Gastrointestinal Physiology

Eugene Trowers • Marc Tischler

Gastrointestinal Physiology

A Clinical Approach

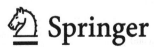 Springer

Eugene Trowers, MD, MPH
Department of Internal Medicine
The University of Arizona
Tucson, AZ, USA

Marc Tischler, BA, MS, PhD
Department of Chemistry and Biochemistry
The University of Arizona
Tucson, AZ, USA

ISBN 978-3-319-07163-3   ISBN 978-3-319-07164-0 (eBook)
DOI 10.1007/978-3-319-07164-0
Springer Cham Heidelberg New York Dordrecht London

Library of Congress Control Number: 2014941602

Printed on acid-free paper

Springer is part of Springer Science+Business Media (www.springer.com)

Preface

This book was designed for those readers specializing in GI as in clerkships, electives, residencies, and beyond. The book provides a focused review of gastro-intestinal physiological principles presented in easy-to-read language. Mastery of the material is tested in multiple ways in real time. Key reasons for reading this book include:

- Practical guide to GI physiology.
- Promotes hands on learning.
- Integrated systems approach for the eight subareas of GI system.
- Easy-to-read format.
- USMLE style questions interspersed throughout chapters prepare readers for in-service, board, and recertification exams.
- Cases formatted as the reader will see them on the wards or clinics.
- Normal range of lab values provided within the body of the case.
- Key concepts highlighted throughout the text in boxes and summarized in one place.
- Unique quick reference tables—"Diseases Affecting the GI tract" and "Neo-plasms of the GI tract"—excellent test prep aids.
- Unique Connecting-the-Dots segments present an illustrative case to reinforce learning in real time.

Allied health, nursing professionals, and trainees who treat patients with gastro-intestinal problems will also find this book useful. For gastroenterology fellows and others involved in advanced training in gastrointestinal diseases, this book may serve as a primer upon which they can build their knowledge as they investigate the more intricate areas of the discipline.

Our book utilizes newer adult learning strategies in medical education. We make connections to a student's life whether at work or in the classroom by presenting relevant cases which are critical in providing a forum in which the student can apply acquired knowledge, skills, and attitudes. Practice is the best way for students to truly gain mastery of a subject or concept.

Despite the use of clinical vignettes and scenarios, this is a physiology book and not a pathophysiology book. We do not delve into certain diseases, tests, or treatments, unless by doing so we further the understanding of gastrointestinal physiology. There are a number of outstanding formal texts that detail nonclinical mechanisms. This book, however, was written for present and future practitioners caring for today's patients and who need to build upon a solid clinical foundation.

In summary, this book is ideal for the students/practitioners of clinical GI physiology who need to review key concepts in order to understand what is going on with their patients and to ace USMLE or other board exams.

Tucson, AZ   Eugene Trowers
Tucson, AZ   Marc Tischler

Contents

Chapter 1
Clinical Gastrointestinal Physiology: A Systems Approach

1.1 Introduction

Physiology students often request integration of the material being taught. Naturally students want the concepts they are learning to "fit together." In fact, in order for information to be relevant and beneficial, it is critical to provide a solid framework upon which concepts can be hung. Upon learning that you were going to study gastrointestinal physiology, perhaps your initial thought was: "I will be studying the stomach and the intestines." Despite the fact that the stomach and intestines play an important role in gastrointestinal functions, they do not account for the entire tale. Rather, one needs to examine the *system* that is accountable for the movement of nutrients into and out of the body.

Gastrointestinal fellows and residents can err in taking care of patients with digestive diseases if they focus only on the stomach or intestines when analyzing the patient's problems. The gastrointestinal system consists of all the components required to transport nutrients from the external environment down the digestive tract, across the intestinal epithelial cells and into the blood, and for the excretion of waste. Primary elements of this system involve muscles and supporting structures, the brain–gut axis, and secretory and nutrient exchange components.

Muscles play a critical role in the generation of intestinal contractions and motility. Without muscles, the esophagus, stomach, and intestines would be rendered useless. Likewise the brain and nervous system play vital roles in the modification of gastrointestinal motility and functions. In the absence of this brain–gut regulation, the gastrointestinal tract muscles would not perform in a well-coordinated fashion. An integrated systems approach holds the solution to understanding gastrointestinal function in normal and altered conditions. Content of the chapters will demonstrate how the various components of the system relate.

E. Trowers and M. Tischler, *Gastrointestinal Physiology*,
DOI 10.1007/978-3-319-07164-0_1, © Springer International Publishing Switzerland 2014

1.2   Summary of Key Learning Tools

Objectives: The abstract of each chapter presents what readers should be able to know or do at the end of the chapter. On finishing the chapter, readers should have obtained certain knowledge, skills, and attitudes.

    Reality checks: Thought questions are interspersed throughout the text to enable mastery of key concepts in real time as opposed to waiting for the end of the chapter.

    Case in point: This tool lays out cases in the way readers will see them when reading a chart—chief complaint, history, physical exam, labs. Questions are posed to evaluate readers' assessments and/or plans.

    Connecting-the-Dots: Illustrative cases facilitating the understanding and retention of important clinical physiologic principles.

    Recall points: Key concepts are highlighted throughout the text to foster retention.

    Summary points: Key concepts are summarized in one place with a user friendly review aid.

    USMLE style review questions: These questions test readers' acquisition of knowledge, skills, and attitudes.

    Answer Keys: At the end of each chapter answer keys are provided for reality checks, Case in Point, Connecting-the-Dots, and review questions.

    Appendix: This section will provide three tables—"Diseases affecting the GI tract," "Neoplasms of the GI tract," and "Clinical laboratory tests" to serve as a unique quick reference and as a user friendly aid for last minute board preparations.

1.3   Value of the Learning Tools

Conceptual thinking is the hallmark of the science of physiology. To recognize how and why the body functions and responds to the disturbances of disease, one must understand physiology. The goal of this book is to emphasize an appreciation of basic physiological concepts versus rote memorization of isolated facts. The reader should grasp certain physiological principles and apply them to novel situations. Hence, when encountering a patient with different alterations in gastrointestinal function, you will be better poised to understand the basis for the patient's problems and what needs to be corrected to remedy the problem. The intent is to expose the healthcare provider-in-training to fundamental principles that are useful in treating patients and which will lay the groundwork for more advanced study in the future. Thus we have chosen to focus on clinical physiology.

    Careful study of animal models and patients contributed significantly to the science of physiology. Those observations generated hypotheses to account for the results. Sometimes the hypotheses underwent rigorous examination and modification as needed. In other cases, physicians must operate empirically because proof may be lacking. This lack of certainty in all settings may be a source of annoyance for those who require absolute answers. Conceivably, if an area of uncertainty attracts your interest, you may decide later in life to conduct further inquiries and experiments that may elucidate a better understanding of how the human body works. Meanwhile, your understanding can be challenged with USMLE style questions and scenarios.

Digestion and absorption are fundamental processes. The study of gastrointestinal physiology is relevant to the study of all medical specialties from medicine to psychiatry. An understanding of nutrient exchange, as well as the matching of absorption and digestion of carbohydrates, proteins, and lipids, is vital for the practicing physician. The events that can disrupt the nutrient exchange are legion and may involve any medical specialty. The coordination of gastrointestinal tract function by the "brain–gut axis" (the special interaction between the automatic and voluntary regulation of gastrointestinal functions) is another important topic for practitioners, as it creates a deeper understanding of a patient's symptoms and behavior. As a healthcare practitioner, internist, surgeon, or psychiatrist, you may encounter a patient with anxiety, diarrhea, or a constellation of other symptoms that are best understood in the framework of gastrointestinal physiology. Individual chapters will demonstrate how the various components of the gastrointestinal system relate.

1.4   Recall Points

1.4.1   Components of the Gastrointestinal System: Brain–Gut Axis; Gastrointestinal Secretion; Nutrient Exchange

The *brain–gut axis* coordinates control of GI motor functions. This axis includes the central nervous system (CNS), the enteric nervous system (ENS), and the enteroendocrine cells. The *gastrointestinal secretion* component consists of assorted structures, which carry out the secretory function of the gastrointestinal system and are listed below.

The secretory cells, glands, intestinal epithelia, and supporting structures are essential for the secretion of biological products involved in multiple digestive processes. For example, mucous helps to lubricate food boluses and facilitate the transport of nutrients. Bicarbonate secreted by the pancreas establishes a favorable environment in which pancreatic enzymes can function. Cholera toxin produces a rampant secretory diarrhea, which can lead to severe volume contraction of the vasculature and electrolyte disturbance if left uncorrected. Finally, the *nutrient exchange* component (the intestinal epithelia, supporting structures, and circulatory apparatus) is the site of exchange of energy sources that are critical for effective and efficient metabolism.

An overview of anatomy of the digestive system, emphasizing the function of key anatomic structures, is provided in Chap. 2. The book then investigates the role of the brain–gut axis in coordinating GI movement and how multiple factors contribute to the control of gastrointestinal motility in Chap. 3. The contents of Chap. 4 focus on gastrointestinal secretion, its controlling factors, and the interplay of the brain–gut axis. Nutrient exchange is covered in Chap. 5. The brain–gut axis' role in digestion and absorption is presented in terms of digestion-related molecules which either directly attack nutrients or work through cell-regulatory effects. The subject matter in Chap. 6 examines key topics concerning the physiology of the liver, gallbladder, and pancreas. Water and electrolyte physiology, which plays an important role in nutrient exchange and gastrointestinal secretion, is considered in Chap. 7. Finally, Chap. 8 integrates what the reader has learned and makes links to the future study of pathophysiology via the evaluation of select motility disorders. You will continually be brought back to the triad of the gastrointestinal system framework—brain–gut axis, gastrointestinal secretion, and nutrient exchange—so that you can see how the individual parts mesh together.

Considering the volume of information presented to physicians today, students and house officers need to determine which portion is essential for mastery. Trainees want to determine, "Why do I need to know this?" For the purposes of this book, the answer to this question is twofold. First, and most obviously, this information will assist you in the care of current and future patients. Second, by building a solid physiological knowledge base you will be able to assimilate new knowledge concerning human physiology and disease states which you will encounter in the future.

Placing the study of gastrointestinal physiology in the clinical context facilitates your appreciation of its relevance. The aim is to clarify and reinforce these integrated concepts. The "Connecting-the-Dots" brief clinical vignette at the end of a chapter illustrates several of the key principles found in the chapter and augment important concepts. Readers are more likely to read and attempt to understand material which they find clinically relevant.

Students of physiology must think critically and the goal of teachers should be to help students do so. To grasp physiological concepts and ultimately help patients, you must be able to think critically and apply learned material to new situations. Rote memorization of facts provides little assistance when you need to answer physiological questions. Therefore a deeper understanding of physiology must be acquired through manipulating the concepts and becoming very familiar with them. That goal is achieved by using a more conceptual approach rather than a quantitative one to facilitate mastery of key principles. Calculations and equations presented focus on those encountered in clinical practice. In addition, several learning tools will enhance your development of a deeper understanding of concepts critical to thinking like a clinical physiologist.

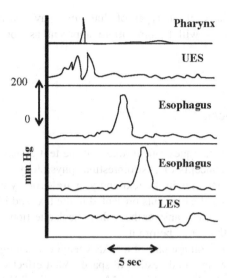

Fig. 1.1 Manometry and muscle contractions. After swallowing notice the pressure complex beginning in the pharynx that gradually closes off the upper esophageal sphincter (UES). The food bolus moves down the esophagus toward the lower esophageal sphincter (LES). LES relaxation commences with the initiation of the swallow and remains relaxed until the bolus reaches the distal esophagus so that it can empty into the stomach. Once the bolus exits the distal esophagus, the LES closes and its pressure returns to its sphincteric level

1.5 Figures

An array of illustrations is included in the text to provide multiple opportunities to work with the concepts presented here. These figures and diagrams allow the reader to manipulate physiological variables over a range of conditions to better understand a concept or principle. You can virtually create experiments by changing conditions and predicting outcomes. These learning opportunities augment the text especially for visual learners and are employed to engross your senses in the learning encounter.

In the case of complex figures, you should first focus on one aspect of the figure, then try to integrate ensuing aspects to develop an understanding of the full picture. In essence, approach the complex figure as a puzzle, piece by piece until the completed picture becomes obvious. As a food bolus moves down the esophagus, one can see an illustrative picture of the contraction and relaxation of the involved upper digestive tract muscles captured by a manometry transducer (Fig. 1.1). How do these opposing forces interact to effectively transport the bolus down the esophagus toward the stomach? What types of manometric changes should you expect to see if the upper digestive tract muscles are compromised in certain ways? Alternatively, if you see a manometric tracing with certain alterations, what types of physiological problems should be expected in the affected patient? These are the types of questions you will need to ask yourself when viewing the diagrams and its associated text. Initially, these types of diagrams may appear challenging, but the illustrated concepts will become more apparent as you work through the chapters.

1.6   Reality Check

Inclusion of reality check questions throughout the text assists the reader to work with principles and concepts of gastrointestinal physiology. These thought questions appear at key junctures in the text and you are strongly encouraged to work through them to master the concepts presented in the text and illustrated figures up to that point. When unable to answer the reality check question, you should stop and review the material that came before it.

   Reality check 1-1: You are part of a NASA team evaluating the effects of zero gravity upon swallowing and digestion in space. What effect would you expect to see when an astronaut eats a meal in the Mir space station? Why?

   Answers to thought questions are found at the end of the chapters.

1.7   Review Questions

Review questions based on short clinical vignettes appear at the end of the chapters and allow you to self-assess your learning. Answers to these review questions can be found at the end of each chapter.

1.8   Connecting-the-Dots

Reading through the chapters, you will learn a variety of facts and principles about the digestive system. Each chapter ends with a section entitled "Connecting-the-Dots," which will enable you to think conceptually and determine how the information presented in the chapter can be used to analyze a patient's problem. Clinical vignettes presented in these sections raise diagnostic and treatment questions. Because this is a physiology and not a pathophysiology text you are not expected to have knowledge of specific disease processes. However, it is very beneficial to learn how physiological concepts can be utilized to solve everyday patient problems. Despite the fact that you have just begun to explore the world of gastrointestinal physiology, consider the following illustrative case:

A 24-year-old medical student comes to the infirmary complaining of burning mid-sternal chest pain. She states that exacerbation of the pain occurs when she bends over to tie her shoes as well assuming a supine position. In addition, the patient states that eating chocolates, peppermints, and drinking alcoholic beverages worsens the pain. The patient states that when she takes antacid medications such as proton pump inhibitors, she experiences complete alleviation of her pain. The physical examination reveals no abnormal findings concerning the heart, lungs, or abdomen. Hemogram, chemistry profile, amylase, lipase, chest X-ray, abdominal plain films, and ECG are unremarkable. What part or parts of the gastrointestinal system are not functioning correctly to account for the patient's heartburn?

1.9   Summary Points

Each chapter concludes with a list of in a nutshell summary points. These points present a succinct review of the high yield concepts covered in the text. Reviewing the learning objectives contained in the abstract at the beginning of the chapter, as well as the summary points and review questions at the end, will facilitate evaluation of your comprehension of the concepts covered in the text.

- The study of gastrointestinal physiology depends upon an understanding that effective and efficient nutrient exchange requires the interaction of different components of the gastrointestinal system. One does not transport and exchange nutrients via the gut alone.
- The major components of the gastrointestinal system include the brain–gut axis, the ENS, the enteroendocrine cells, and the gastrointestinal secretion component.
- You should work through all thought questions and Figures to master the concepts outlined in this book.

1.10   Answer to Connecting-the-Dots

The patient shows evidence of problems with gastroesophageal reflux. As depicted in Fig. 1.1, intraesophageal pressure is less than lower esophageal sphincter (LES) pressure, which in turn exceeds the gastric pressure. Bending over or assuming the supine position induces an increase in intra-abdominal pressure that in turn potentiates reflux of gastric contents. Alcohol consumption or ingestion of chocolate and peppermint decreases LES pressure resulting in the reflux of stomach acid into the esophagus and the sensation of burning chest pain. By the time you complete reading this book, you will be able to ascertain the physiological concepts and principles which underlie a patient's symptoms and physical findings. In this way you will develop a deeper appreciation for the wonders of gastrointestinal physiology.

1.11   Answers to Reality Check

Reality check 1-1: The effect of zero gravity upon various organ systems is a question of great concern for NASA scientists. One might theorize that it might take a longer period of time for a food bolus to travel down the esophagus when unaided by gravity. However, gravity produces little effect on swallowing and digestion in general. In contrast, zero gravity creates a more pronounced effect on circulation and causes calcium to leach out of bones.

Suggested Reading

Costanzo LS. Physiology. 4th ed. Philadelphia: Saunders; 2010. Chapter 8, Gastrointestinal physiology; p. 327–78.

Kahrilas PJ, Pandolfino JE. Esophageal motor function. In: Yamada T, Alpers DH, Kalloo AN, Kaplowitz N, Owyang C, Powell DW, editors. Textbook of gastroenterology. 5th ed. Oxford: Wiley-Blackwell; 2009. Chapter 9.

Kibble JD, Halsey CR. The big picture: medical physiology. New York: McGraw Hill; 2009. Chapter 7, Gastrointestinal physiology; p. 259–306.

Chapter 2
Form and Function: The Physiological Implications of the Anatomy of the Gastrointestinal System

2.1 Introduction

The digestive system consists of a series of organs and glands that process ingested food by physical and chemical means to provide the body absorbable nutrients and to excrete waste products. In humans, this system includes the alimentary canal, and associated glands which run from the mouth to the anus, plus the hormones and enzymes which assist in digestion. The digestive system is considered in light of its major roles, not only with respect to nutrient exchange but also in regard to its support of other bodily activities and maintenance of homeostasis.

2.2 Digestive System Requirements: Form Meets Function

2.2.1 Absorptive and Secretory Mucosa

The gut wall comprises four concentric layers as you move from the lumen toward the outer surface: (1) mucosa, (2) submucosa, (3) muscularis propria, and (4) serosa (Fig. 2.1).

The inner surface of the intestines is arranged into longitudinal folds (*plicae circulares* or *Kerckring folds*), which in turn give rise to finger-like projections called *villi* (Fig. 2.1). Epithelial cells and mucus secreting *goblet cells* cover the surface of the villi. The mucus secreted by the goblet cells helps to lubricate food stuffs and facilitate movement in the intestinal tract. The *apical surface* of the villi gives rise to *microvilli*, which increase the absorptive surface area (Fig. 2.1). When viewed with a light microscope, the microvillar surface has a *brush border* appearance. Cells located toward the tips of the villi absorb intestinal contents and those located at the base of the villi or crypts secrete fluids and electrolytes.

The intestinal mucosa is designed to absorb nutrients and fluids via two main paths: (1) a *transcellular path* in which the substance must cross the apical or brush

E. Trowers and M. Tischler, *Gastrointestinal Physiology*,
DOI 10.1007/978-3-319-07164-0_2, © Springer International Publishing Switzerland 2014

Fig. 2.1 Cross section of the gut wall highlighting the four concentric layers from the lumen toward the outer surface. The insets show details for a villus and the microvilli on an enterocyte (absorptive intestinal cell) on the villus

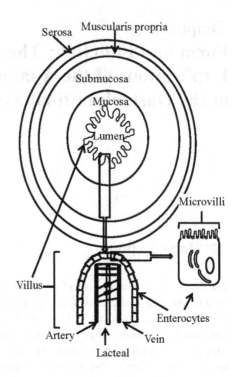

border of the intestinal cell, enter into the cell, and then exit the cell across the basolateral border and (2) a *paracellular path* where substances cross *tight junctions* between adjacent intestinal cells, through the intercellular spaces and into the blood (Fig. 2.2). Mechanisms of absorption and secretion will be discussed in later chapters. As you will see, the GI tract muscles, nerves, and vasculature ultimately act to facilitate the functions of the absorptive and secretory mucosa.

Reality check 2-1: A tennis superstar has recently been diagnosed with Sjogren's disease, a chronic autoimmune disease in which a patient's white blood cells attack his/her moisture-producing glands. What type of an effect would you expect concerning swallowing during a long hot match during the US Open? What would you expect if he/she later is overwhelmed with emotion after a tremendously difficult victory?

2.2.2   Muscles

In general, form and function of the human body are closely related. Nature tends to select features which provide survival advantage.

The following layers are seen in a typical cross section of the gut wall when viewed from the outer surface toward the inward surface: (1) serosa, (2) longitudinal muscle, (3) circular muscle, (4) submucosa, and (5) mucosa (Fig. 2.1).

Fig. 2.2 Mechanisms of nutrient absorption in the small intestine. The transcellular pathway may involve either passive permeability (*left*) or carrier-mediated transport (*middle*) from the apical surface at the lumen side or the basolateral surface at the blood side. The paracellular pathway (*right*) crosses tight junctions between adjacent cells

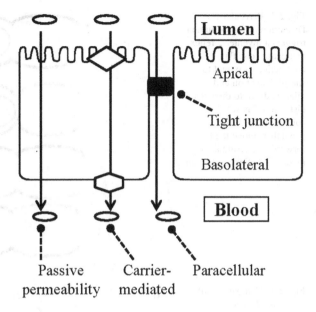

Passive permeability   Carrier-mediated   Paracellular

The *muscularis mucosae* consists of sparse bundles of smooth muscle fibers located between the *submucosal plexus* and the *lamina propria*. The smooth muscle present in the muscularis mucosae is responsible for movement in the mucosal layer of the gut wall. The pressure necessary to propel luminal contents down the GI tract in the process of *peristalsis* actually comes from circular muscle contraction above a point of distension and concurrent relaxation of this muscle layer below the luminal contents (Fig. 2.3). Contraction of the longitudinal muscle during this process shortens the distance over which the circular muscle contraction has to travel in order to move the contents forward.

Whereas striated muscle contraction is under conscious control, smooth muscle contraction is involuntary. Imagine a GI tract under complete conscious control. For peristalsis to move a food bolus along the entire gut one would have to consciously initiate and maintain the effort. That would literally require a lot of thought and would be very inefficient. Fortunately, gut wall smooth muscles have some unique properties which enable them to perform their principal functions. The smooth muscle cells contain actin and myosin filaments in an arrangement which is not as ordered as the sarcomeres of skeletal muscle. Intestinal muscle cells do not actually appear "smooth" when viewed under a light microscope (Fig. 2.4a); they simply lack the striations seen in skeletal muscle (Fig. 2.4b) and, therefore, have a more uniform appearance.

The GI tract comprises unitary smooth muscle which has a high degree of electrochemical coupling between adjacent cells because of the presence of many gap junctions. Because of this special arrangement, stimulation of one cell causes the group of connected cells to contract simultaneously as a *syncytium*. Some smooth muscles (e.g., those found in the esophageal body, small intestine, and

Fig. 2.3 Peristalsis. Distention of the GI lumen triggers a myenteric reflex that causes circular contraction proximal to the site of distention and dilation distal to the site of distention. These contractions, termed peristalsis, move the bolus forward, triggering another myenteric reflex, and so on

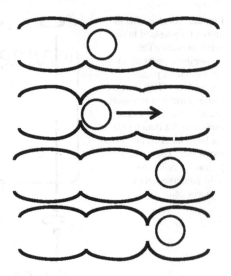

Fig. 2.4 Comparison of structure of muscle. (**a**) Structure of smooth muscle: spindle-shaped with single nuclei. (**b**) Structure of skeletal muscle: striated and multinucleated

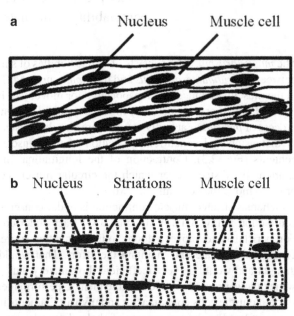

gastric antrum) contract and relax in a few seconds (phasic contractions). Smooth muscles found in the *lower esophageal sphincter* (LES), ileocecal valve, and anal sphincters may contract over minutes or hours (tonic contractions). The type of contraction is determined by the smooth muscle cell and is independent of neural or hormonal input.

Unitary smooth muscle exhibits slow waves (i.e., spontaneous pacemaker activity) and represents undulations of 5–15 mV in the smooth muscle membrane

Fig. 2.5 Interstitial cells of Cajal and their processes form multiple connections with adjacent smooth muscle cells

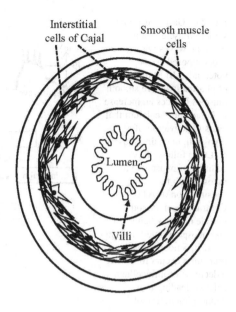

potential. These periodic membrane depolarizations and repolarizations are major determinants of the phasic nature of GI smooth muscle contraction. The rate of slow waves and subsequent rhythmic contractions is 3 per minute in the stomach, 12 per minute in the duodenum, and 9 per minute in the terminal ileum. Slow wave activity is due to ionic currents initiated via the interactions of the *interstitial cells of Cajal* (ICCs) with smooth muscle cells (Fig. 2.5). Slow wave generation involves the cyclic opening of calcium channels during depolarization and the opening of potassium channels subsequently during repolarization. Spike potentials are true action potentials which are superimposed on slow waves. When the resting membrane potential of the GI smooth muscle becomes more positive than approximately -40 mV, then spike potentials occur and smooth muscle contraction is initiated (Fig. 2.6a).

In phasically active muscles, stimulation induces a rise in intracellular calcium, which induces phosphorylation of the light chain of myosin (Fig. 2.6b). ATP splits and the muscle contracts as the phosphorylated myosin interacts with actin. When calcium concentration decreases, myosin is dephosphorylated and relaxation occurs. In tonically active muscles, contraction can be maintained at low levels of phosphorylation and ATP utilization. Intestinal smooth muscle action potentials are largely mediated by the inward movement of Ca^{2+} rather than Na^+. This difference has important ramifications with regard to the classes of pharmacologic agents that can suppress intestinal motility (e.g., calcium channel blockers like verapamil) without significantly affecting skeletal muscle function because skeletal (voluntary) muscle contraction is controlled principally by the central nervous system (CNS).

The two major types of movements in the GI tract are (1) peristalsis or *propulsive movements* and (2) mixing or *segmentation movements* (Fig. 2.7). GI peristalsis (anywhere except the skeletal muscle region of the esophagus) requires an intact

Fig. 2.6 Gastrointestinal smooth muscle function. (**a**) Slow waves with superimposed action potentials. (**b**) Stimulation of phasically active smooth muscles induces an increase in intracellular calcium that leads to activation of myosin light chain kinase (MLCK) followed by addition of phosphate to myosin with the consumption of ATP. Contraction of smooth muscle occurs when actin and phosphorylated myosin interact. Smooth muscle relaxation occurs following a decrease of intracellular calcium leading to dephosphorylation of myosin

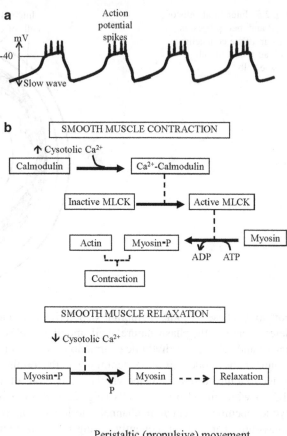

Fig. 2.7 Comparison of peristaltic contractions with mixing contractions in the small bowel. Peristaltic contractions propel the chyme in a caudad direction. Segmentation contractions mix the chyme

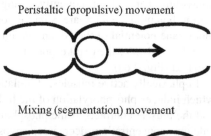

Peristaltic (propulsive) movement

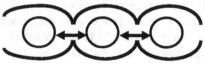

Mixing (segmentation) movement

and functional myenteric plexus; the contribution to this process made by the respective muscle layers involved is their ability to either contract (above) or relax (below) a point of distension, but this is coordinated by the myenteric plexus and cannot occur in its absence. Physical stretching of unitary smooth muscle may cause smooth muscle excitation but this excitation by itself does not initiate a peristaltic wave (just a contraction) and, again, this phenomenon cannot be propagated without the coordinating influence of the myenteric plexus. However, once a peristaltic wave is propagated unconsciously, it can be propagated with much greater efficiency which frees our brains to ponder other weighty physiology questions. When a bolus of food enters the esophagus, a primary peristaltic wave of contraction of esophageal muscle passes from the oral to the gastric end. If this primary wave does not cause the bolus to exit from the esophagus, then a secondary peristaltic wave occurs in an attempt to move the food bolus. The LES must be able to relax for the food bolus to exit the esophagus. In addition, the LES must remain a competent sphincter in order to prohibit the reflux of gastric contents into the esophagus.

The relationships between the myenteric plexus, GI smooth muscle, and coordinated motor activity are crucial to understanding the pathophysiological basis of certain motility disorders of the intestines. Patients with primary disorders of small intestinal motility may appear to have intestinal obstruction due to decreased or absent motility and bowel distention. Patients with idiopathic intestinal pseudo-obstruction have a derangement of smooth muscle cells that results in delayed transit or transient ileus or apparent paralysis. Metabolic abnormalities, e.g., the depletion of potassium or administration of drugs such as anticholinergics, decrease neural transmission via the *enteric nervous system* (ENS) resulting in decreased small intestinal motility.

Factors that control colonic motility are not completely understood. However, as is the case in the stomach and small intestine, the following factors are involved in the control of colonic motility: (1) ICCs, (2) properties of smooth muscles, (3) the ENS, and (4) locally released or circulating chemicals. *Hirschsprung's disease* is a developmental disorder of the ENS characterized by an absence of ganglion cells in the distal colon. The enteric neurons in the distal colon and internal anal sphincter seem to be predominantly inhibitory because when they are destroyed or absent the colon is tonically contracted resulting in decreased colonic motility and constipation. Surgical removal of the diseased segment allows normal colonic contractions to occur.

Reality check 2-2: Scleroderma is a rare, progressive connective tissue disease that involves hardening and tightening of the skin and supportive tissues that normally provide the supportive framework for your body. What type of esophageal dysmotility findings would you expect?

Connecting-the-Dots 2-1

A 54-year-old male comes to the emergency room complaining of right lower quadrant abdominal pain. Preoperatively he was diagnosed with acute appendicitis. At operation an inflamed and perforated diverticulum of the cecum was found. The surgeon performed a cecostomy (surgically constructed drainage procedure of the cecum). After 3 weeks the cecostomy

(continued)

still did not function. During this time, the patient lost large volumes (5–7 L) of gastric secretion daily. Glucose, physiological saline, and plasma were given via IV. Also during this period he developed bloating, constipation, and nausea—all symptoms of decreased intestinal motility. At the end of the 3 weeks, the patient's peripheral reflexes were nearly absent but he was not paralyzed. The patient's serum chloride was 81 mmol/L (normal: 95–108). What was the likely factor that caused the decreased intestinal motility and the mechanism that led to this complication?

2.2.3 Gastrointestinal Smooth Muscle Tonic Contractions

Some GI smooth muscles may undergo tonic contractions as well as, or instead of, rhythmical contractions. Tonic contractions are not associated with the basic electrical rhythm of the slow waves. Tonic contractions occur continuously, often increasing or decreasing in intensity and frequently lasting for several minutes or hours. Tonic contractions may be caused by continuous repetitive spike potentials or by hormones or other factors which cause continuous partial depolarization of smooth muscle membrane without giving rise to action potentials. Continuous movement of Ca^{2+} into the cell interior via a mechanism other than changes in the membrane potential is another cause of tonic contraction in GI smooth muscle. Examples of smooth muscle digestive system sphincters include the LES, the pyloric sphincter at the gastric emptying point, the ileocecal valve, and the internal anal sphincter which is a thickening of the inner circular muscle layer.

2.2.4 Nervous Innervation: General Features

While the brain-gut axis modulates intestinal function, the bulk of the afferent–efferent activity occurs via intrinsic rather than extrinsic innervation. The GI system is similar to the cardiovascular, endocrine, and respiratory systems because it can function without the need for conscious control. The autonomic nervous system (ANS) includes the ENS, which constitutes the intrinsic innervation of the gut and the sympathetic and parasympathetic divisions which provide extrinsic innervation to the intestine (Fig. 2.8a). The ENS consists of the *myenteric (Auerbach's) plexus* and the *submucosal (Meissner's) plexus* (Fig. 2.8b). Auerbach's plexus is located between the inner circular and outer longitudinal muscle layers which control gut wall motility. Meissner's plexus lies in the submucosa and controls secretion and blood flow. The enteric plexuses comprise nerve cell bodies, axons, dendrites, and nerve endings. The neuronal processes of the

Fig. 2.8 The autonomic innervation of the gastrointestinal system and the structure of the enteric wall. (**a**) General overview showing the relationships of the CNS (central nervous system) and ANS (autonomic nervous system) with the ENS (enteric nervous system). (**b**) Interaction of the myenteric and submucosal plexuses with smooth muscle of the intestinal wall. The myenteric plexus controls gut motility and the submucosal plexus controls secretions and blood flow

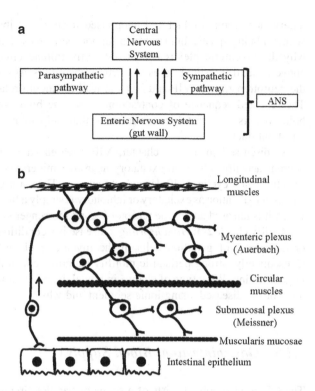

enteric plexuses innervate target cells, e.g., secretory, absorptive, and smooth muscle cells, and make connection to sensory receptors and make connections with other neurons both inside and outside the plexus. Hence, integration of various activities can be achieved entirely through the ENS.

The role of neurotransmitters in the ANS: Several neurotransmitters are localized in specific pathways within the ANS. *Acetylcholine (ACh)* is the neurotransmitter found in many of the extrinsic nervous system, preganglionic efferent fibers, and exerts its action on neurons found in the prevertebral ganglia as well as the intrinsic nervous system. *Norepinephrine (NE)* is often found in the postganglionic efferent nerves of the sympathetic nervous system and frequently exerts its effect on the ENS neurons.

Neurotransmitters such as ACh, nitric oxide (NO), vasoactive intestinal peptide (VIP), somatostatin, and serotonin have been localized to interneurons in the ENS. VIP and NO have been found localized to nerves that are inhibitory to the muscle versus ACh and substance P which have been localized to nerves that are excitatory to muscle. An understanding of the neuronal circuits intrinsic to the intestine is helpful in understanding the mechanism of certain GI motility disorders such as Hirschsprung's disease (described above) that primarily affects the rectum and left colon. In the aganglionic segments, NO and VIP neural transmission is ablated resulting in the aganglionic segment's failure to relax and remain contracted. In addition, the extrinsic parasympathetic, cholinergic, and sympathetic adrenergic innervations remain intact and unopposed further contributing to the aganglionic segment being spastic and unable to support peristalsis. This scenario also explains why the myenteric plexus can concurrently initiate circular muscle contraction above a small intestinal bolus via neurotransmitters ACh and Substance P, while the neurotransmitters VIP and NO can lead to smooth relaxation below the bolus. The repeated sequence of contraction above the bolus and relaxation below the bolus results in peristaltic contractions that help to move the bolus down the intestinal tract.

As discussed in a later chapter, VIP released from submucosal secretomotor neurons actually acts as an excitatory neurotransmitter when it stimulates crypt cell secretion via a cyclic AMP-dependent pathway. Thus, a neurotransmitter is just that and its classification as excitatory or inhibitory is simply a function of the structure onto which it is released and/or the receptor-second messenger system that it then affects.

Reality check 2-3: *Hirschsprung's* disease is a condition characterized by a lack or deficiency of ganglion cells in the myenteric plexus in the sigmoid colon. Consequently, strong peristaltic motility cannot occur in this diseased area of the large intestine. What type of change in bowel diameter would you expect above the level of the diseased aganglionic segment and why?

2.2.5   Gastrointestinal Blood Supply

The GI blood supply consists of a series of parallel circuits that allow blood to be diverted away or directed to specific areas without altering the entire blood supply to the gut as a whole (Fig. 2.9). The splanchnic circulation refers to all organs fed by the celiac (stomach), superior mesenteric (right colon, part of transverse colon, and small intestine), and inferior mesenteric (left colon) arteries. The blood from these organs then collects into the portal vein to drain to the liver. One-third of the total blood volume in a resting person is distributed in the splanchnic circulation. Hence, the splanchnic circulation has a reservoir function greater than any other body region.

Absorption of nutrients takes place in the small intestine. The superior mesenteric artery comes from the aorta to supply the jejunum and ileum (Fig. 2.9) via a series of intercommunicating arcades which travel through the mesentery. Small arteries penetrate the intestinal wall and ultimately supply the capillary network of the intestinal villus tip. In close proximity to the arterial capillary, the venous capillary blood leaves the villus and returns via the intestinal veins and corresponding superior mesenteric vein (Fig. 2.10).

The splenic vein joins with the superior mesenteric vein to form the portal vein which will drain to the liver sinusoids where the reticuloendothelial and hepatic cells absorb and temporally store up to three quarters of all absorbed nutrients. The majority of fat-based nutrients are absorbed into the intestinal lymphatics and then directed to the circulating blood by the thoracic duct, bypassing the liver. The hepatic veins deliver blood from the liver to the vena cava and ultimately to the right atrium.

Fig. 2.9 Splanchnic circulation. Several arteries carry blood from the aorta to the stomach, spleen, pancreas, small intestine, and large intestine. The blood from these organs collects in the portal vein that drains into the liver

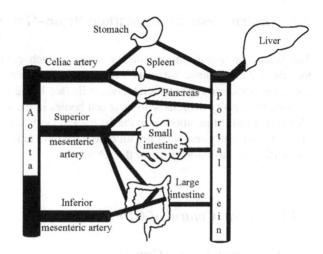

Fig. 2.10 Microcirculation to intestinal villi

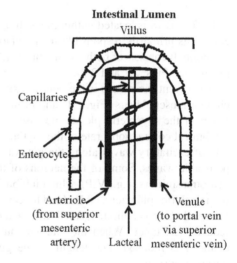

Reality check 2-4: A 76-year-old retired GI physiology professor is undergoing emergency abdominal angiography because of massive lower GI bleeding. You observe a blush of contrast spurting from a rent in the superior mesenteric artery. Which portion of the patient's colon should be resected?

2.2.6 Recall Points

Digestive System Requirements
- Absorptive and secretory mucosa
- Muscles (inner circular, outer longitudinal)
- Nervous innervation (intrinsic, extrinsic); blood supply

2.3   Gastrointestinal Regulation: Brain–Gut Axis

The *brain–gut axis* is the regulatory system which controls GI functions and includes the interconnection of the central nervous system (CNS; brain and spinal cord), the ENS, and the enteroendocrine cells (see Fig. 2.8).

Afferent sensory neurons with their cell bodies in the submucosal or myenteric plexus transmit information from the GI tract to the brain for processing. Intrinsic efferent axons carry neural information from the CNS to the ENS. Extrinsic efferent axons carry neural information to the ANS.

2.3.1   Neural Control of GI Function

2.3.1.1   Intrinsic Nervous Control

ENS: The ENS is located within the wall of the GI tract from the esophagus to the anus. It is primarily responsible for regulating movement within the GI tract and secretion. It consists of both the myenteric (Auerbach's) plexus and the submucosal plexus (see Figs. 2.1 and 2.8).

The myenteric plexus is the outer plexus that lies between the longitudinal and circular muscle layers (Fig. 2.1) and primarily controls gut motor activity. Stimulation of the myenteric plexus increases gut wall tonic contraction, intensity of rhythmical contractions, rate of the rhythm of contraction, and velocity of conduction of excitatory waves along the gut wall resulting in more rapid movement of peristaltic waves. Some of the neurons of the myenteric plexus secrete inhibitory neurotransmitters (e.g., VIP), which inhibit intestinal sphincter muscles. Inhibition of the pyloric sphincter enables food to leave the stomach with less resistance. If the ileocecal valve is inhibited, small intestinal contents can empty into the colon with reduced resistance. When the circular muscle is stimulated to contract, the gut diameter is reduced. The length of the gut is shortened when the longitudinal muscle contracts.

The submucosal plexus receives sensory signals from mechanoreceptors and chemoreceptors in the GI tract and controls secretion and blood flow within the inner wall of the gut.

2.3.1.2   Neural Control of GI Function: Extrinsic Nervous Control

Parasympathetic Nervous System: The vagus nerve (cranial nerve X) and the pelvic nerve supply parasympathetic innervation to the GI tract. Both of these nerves contain efferent (motor) and afferent (sensory) fibers. The vagus nerve supplies the upper GI tract. The innervations include the striated muscle in the upper third of the esophagus, the wall of the stomach, the small intestine, and the right colon. The vagus nerve provides extrinsic innervation to esophageal striated muscle that is necessary for contractile activity in the skeletal muscle portion. However, it does not serve the same function in the smooth muscle region where the myenteric plexus regulates this activity. Vagovagal reflexes are sensory-motor reflexes carried in the vagus nerve. The lower GI tract, including the striated muscle of the external anal canal, transverse, descending, and sigmoid colon, is innervated by the pelvic nerve.

The parasympathetic nerves are characterized by long preganglionic fibers which synapse in ganglia located in the wall of the GI tract within the myenteric or submucosal plexuses. The parasympathetic postganglionic neurons are classified as either cholinergic or peptidergic.

ACh, the neurotransmitter released from cholinergic neurons, leads to an increase in GI motility and secretions. Peptidergic neurons release one of several different peptides. VIP, when released from the postganglionic peptidergic neuron, results in a decrease in the constriction of GI tract sphincters.

Sympathetic Nervous System: The preganglionic fibers of the sympathetic nervous system originate in the thoracic and lumbar segments of the spinal cord and are generally shorter than those of the parasympathetic nervous system. The preganglionic nerve fibers of the sympathetic nervous system exit in the spinal nerves and in general form synapses in a paired chain of ganglia, which lay outside the GI tract. There are four sympathetic ganglia which serve the GI tract: celiac, superior mesenteric, inferior mesenteric, and hypogastric. These sympathetic post-ganglionic fibers synapse on ganglia in the myenteric and submucosal plexuses or directly innervate smooth muscle, secretory, or endocrine cells. They are adrenergic and secrete norepinephrine, which causes a decrease in GI tract motility and secretions but an increase in the constriction of GI sphincters.

Reality check 2-5: What would you expect to happen to gastrointestinal peristalsis in an individual who is given Atropine (an anticholinergic medication)? Why?

Reality check 2-6: You are evaluating a patient who has suffered a complete C4 cervical cord transection after a motor vehicle accident. What type of bowel movement alteration would you expect and why?

2.3.2 Regulatory Function of Gastrointestinal Peptides

Endocrine (hormones), paracrine agents, and neurotransmitters are peptides that regulate functions in the GI tract (Fig. 2.11). Hormones are peptides secreted by GI endocrine cells into the portal circulation which then pass through the liver and enter the systemic circulation. The hormones are delivered to the receptors of their target cells that may lie within or outside the GI tract. For example, gastrin belongs to the hormone family gastrin–cholecystokinin and is secreted by the G cells of the stomach in response to stomach distention, peptides, and gastrin-releasing peptide (GRP) (Table 2.1). Gastrin secretion results in increased stomach motility, secretion

Fig. 2.11 Comparison of endocrine, paracrine, and neurotransmitter functions

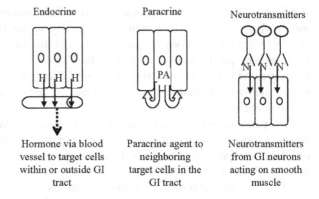

Endocrine	Paracrine	Neurotransmitters
Hormone via blood vessel to target cells within or outside GI tract	Paracrine agent to neighboring target cells in the GI tract	Neurotransmitters from GI neurons acting on smooth muscle

of acid, and increased growth of gastric mucosa. *Cholecystokinin (CCK)*, also belongs to the hormone family Gastrin–CCK and is secreted by the I cells of the duodenum and jejunum in response to fat, amino acids, and small peptides entering the duodenum. CCK secretion stimulates pancreatic enzyme and bicarbonate secretion and leads to contraction of the gallbladder and relaxation of the sphincter of Oddi. CCK also stimulates exocrine pancreas growth and inhibits stomach emptying.

Secretin, a member of the hormone family secretin–glucagon, is secreted by S cells lining the duodenum. Secretion of secretin in the duodenum is stimulated by H^+ as well as by the presence of fatty acids. Release of secretin leads to increased pancreatic and biliary secretion of bicarbonate. Secretin inhibits gastric H^+ secretion as well as the trophic effect of gastrin on the gastric mucosa. VIP is a peptide with close structural homology to secretin. Like secretin, VIP secretes pancreatic bicarbonate which inhibits gastric acid secretion. *Gastric inhibitory peptide (GIP) aka glucose-dependent insulinotrophic peptide*, a member of the hormone family secretin–glucagon, is secreted by duodenal and jejunal mucosal cells. GIP is the only GI hormone that is secreted in response to the three types of nutrients (fats, carbohydrates, and amino acids). GIP stimulates insulin secretion by the beta cells of the pancreas and inhibits gastric acid secretion.

Paracrines are agents released from endocrine cells of the GI tract that diffuse into the interstitial fluid and affect neighboring target cells that possess receptors for the agent. Hence, they act locally and do not enter the systemic circulation. *Somatostatin* and *histamine* are the primary GI paracrine agents. Endocrine cells of the GI mucosa secrete somatostatin in response to decreased luminal pH. Somatostatin strongly inhibits release of most GI hormones and inhibits gastric H^+ secretion. Aside from its paracrine function, somatostatin is secreted by the hypothalamus and by the delta cells of the islets of Langerhans in the pancreas. Histamine is secreted by enteroendocrine cells in the GI mucosa especially in H^+ secreting areas of the stomach. Histamine stimulates gastric acid secretion by activation of parietal cell H_2-type receptors.

Table 2.1 Regulatory functions of peptides secreted by enteroendocrine cells

Hormone	Location produced	Action
Cholecystokinin (CCK)	Peptide hormone produced by I cells in the duodenum and to a lesser extent the jejunum in response to fats, small peptides, and amino acids in the intestine. Release inhibited by somatostatin	Main effect is the contraction of smooth muscle of the gall bladder with increased bile production/secretion and production/secretion of pancreatic enzymes to promote digestion. Along with secretin, regulates rate of stomach emptying and inhibits gastrin release from G cells in the stomach
Enteroglucagon	Mainly terminal ileum and colon from the prohormone preproglucagon	Decreases production of gastric acid by parietal cells and smooth muscle contraction (motility) of the stomach, thereby decreasing gastric emptying
Gastrin	Produced by G-cells in response to presence of undigested proteins, vagal stimulation, distension of the antrum of the stomach, and gastrin-releasing peptide. Inhibited by pH <4 and somatostatin	Stimulates HCl, pepsinogen and intrinsic factor secretion from parietal cells, pepsinogen by chief cells as well as histamine release from enterochromaffin-like cells. Also increases stomach motility (i.e., smooth muscle contraction) and growth of gastric mucosa
Gastric inhibitory peptide (GIP) aka glucose-dependent insulinotropic peptide	Peptide hormone produced in mucosal cells of the duodenum and jejunum. Stimulated by fats, carbohydrates, and amino acids	Decreases gastric acid release by parietal cells as well as smooth muscle contraction (motility) of the stomach. Also increases insulin secretion by pancreatic beta cells and fatty acid metabolism (e.g., milk digestion) by activating lipoprotein lipase
Histamine	Primarily by acid secreting cells of the stomach	Stimulates gastric acid secretion by activation of parietal cell H_2-type receptors
Motilin	Peptide made mainly in the duodenum and jejunum. Secretion stimulus unknown	Increases smooth muscle contraction (fundus, antrum, and gall bladder). Also, stimulates secretion of somatostatin, pancreatic peptide, and pepsinogen
Secretin	Produced by the S-cells in the duodenum. Secretion stimulated by acid or fatty acids in the duodenum	Increased secretion of water and bicarbonate as well as insulin from the pancreas and bile from the liver. Inhibits production of gastrin to reduce

(continued)

Table 2.1 (continued)

Hormone	Location produced	Action
		acidity (pH) entering the duodenum. Lowered pH maximizes activation of pancreatic enzymes secreted into this part of the small intestine. Also enhances secretion of pepsin as well as glucagon, pancreatic polypeptide, and somatostatin
Somatostatin	Produced in endocrine cells of the stomach, intestines, and pancreas	Decreases release of gastrin, CCK, secretin, motilin, VIP, GIP, and enteroglucagon, decreasing stomach secretion and contraction
Vasoactive intestinal peptide (VIP)	Peptide hormone produced in digestive tract and brain	Causes relaxation of smooth muscle (LES, stomach, and gallbladder), stimulates pepsinogen secretion, dilutes bile and pancreatic juice, increases bicarbonate production in the pancreas, decreases gastrin-induced gastric acid secretion, and increases water secretion in intestine

Prostaglandins are eicosanoids that exert paracrine effects on gastric mucosal cells resulting in the antagonism of histamine's stimulation of H^+ secretion by activating a G_i protein that inhibits adenylyl cyclase, thereby lowering cyclic AMP. In addition, prostaglandins enhance submucosal microcirculation. Nonsteroidal anti-inflammatory drugs (NSAIDs) inhibit the effect of prostaglandins. Hence, a patient who consumes NSAIDs experiences uninhibited H^+ secretion and a reduction of the submucosal microcirculation that will lead to the retardation in the healing of peptic ulcer. Similarly, the prostaglandins are prosecretory in the intestine. Patients with *inflammatory bowel disease* (IBD) have inflammatory-related secretory diarrhea. When IBD patients take the salicylate-based NSAIDs, they experience an inhibition of their inflammation-related secretory diarrhea.

Let us briefly examine some examples of how paracrine agents and neurotransmitters may interact. By examining the order in which these substances might be released physiologically and their functions, we can better appreciate their interactions. For example, secretin increases duodenal pH by decreasing acid production, slows gastric activities to emptying and mopping up H^+ ions via pancreatic HCO_3^- secretion. This interaction between the effects of secretin upon gastric acid secretion, gastric emptying, and pancreatic bicarbonate secretion all serve to enhance the digestive function. It is useful to consider functional and structural similarities in attempting to better understand the roles played by GI peptides. VIP and secretin both stimulate pancreatic duct cell HCO_3^-. Interestingly both peptides have nine amino acids that are identical and are classified as members of the secretin family of peptides.

Peptides synthesized in the cell bodies of GI tract neurons are released in response to an action potential in the neuron and act as a neurotransmitter. ACh and NE, two major neurotransmitters, are released into and by the ENS. ACh, secreted by cholinergic neurons, causes contraction of GI wall smooth muscle and the relaxation of GI tract sphincters. In addition, ACh secretion increases salivary, gastric, and pancreatic secretions. NE, secreted by adrenergic neurons, causes relaxation of gut wall smooth muscle as well as contraction of GI sphincters and increased salivary secretion. VIP secretion by neurons of the myenteric and submucosal plexuses results in relaxation of gut smooth muscle. VIP (like secretin) potently stimulates duct cell HCO_3^- secretion, but exerts only a minimal effect on acinar cell enzyme secretion (CCK produces the opposite effect with respect to these cell types). VIP also increases intestinal and pancreatic secretions. *GRP* secretion by neurons of the gastric mucosa increases gastrin secretion. *Substance P* is secreted along with ACh and leads to GI smooth muscle contraction and increased salivary secretion. *Enkephalins* (endogenous opioid peptides) are secreted by mucosal and smooth muscle neurons and cause contraction of gut smooth muscle and decreased intestinal secretion. Opiates in general raise GI smooth muscle tone by suppressing the release of intrinsic inhibitory neurotransmitters thus allowing the inherent excitability of GI smooth muscle to be expressed.

Given that the ENS is called "the little brain" (Fig. 2.8) because it contains all of the neurotransmitters found in the CNS (with the exception of histamine and epinephrine) it would seem much more likely that there will be a region- and function-specific release of a variety of substances that extend well beyond the traditional postganglionic parasympathetic and sympathetic neurotransmitters of simply ACh or NE. For example, in the colon about 70 % of neurally mediated epithelial secretion is atropine resistant, suggesting a major role for at least one other neurotransmitter in this process other than ACh.

Intrinsic Primary Afferent Neurons (IPANs) are neurons that have their cell bodies in the gut wall and whose sensitive endings are in the lamina propria, beneath the mucosal epithelium, in the muscle. 5-Hydroxytryptamine (5-HT) is a potent IPAN stimulant released from mucosal enterochromaffin-like cells that acts as an intermediate in enteric reflexes. When the mucosa is mechanically stimulated, 5-HT is released to elicit motility reflexes. Upon administration of 5-HT antagonists, the motility reflexes will be inhibited.

Kinins are peptides that split from kininogens in areas of inflammation and facilitate the changes in the vasculature associated with inflammation. Kinins also serve as activators of neuronal pain receptors.

2.3.3 Recall Points

Requirements of Gastrointestinal Regulation via Brain–Gut Axis
• Neural control

   – Intrinsic control (ENS)
   – Extrinsic control (parasympathetic and sympathetic nervous systems)

• GI hormones and peptides

Reality check 2-7: Endoscopic retrograde cholangiopancreatography (ERCP) is a procedure performed to diagnose and treat problems of the liver, gallbladder, bile ducts, and pancreas (e.g., gallstones, ductal leaks, and obstruction due to strictures or cancer). ERCP combines the use of a lighted and flexible tube called an endoscope and X-rays. Hence, the physician can see inside the stomach and duodenum and inject the bile and pancreatic ducts with dye which can be seen on X-ray. You are trying to locate where the bile duct enters into the duodenum during an ERCP in a patient who has a gallbladder. Why would the intravenous injection of CCK be helpful?

2.4 Nutrient Exchange

2.4.1 Requirements for Nutrient Exchange

The primary function of the digestive tract is the absorption of nutrients. To accomplish its mission, food must be reduced to more easily absorbable units. The digestive tract contains special anatomical features, which enhance the absorption of nutrients. Most absorption of nutrients occurs in the small intestine that measures ~22 ft. The small intestinal mucosa gives rise to Kerckring folds, which in turn give rise to the villi and microvilli. The end result is a 500–600 % increase in absorptive surface area. Absorption through the GI mucosa takes place primarily via active transport, diffusion, and solvent drag (Fig. 2.2).

2.4.2 Absorption Basics

Seven to eight L of water are absorbed iso-osmotically by diffusion in the small intestine. Imagine if the GI tract did not keep the luminal contents isotonic. In the case of hypertonic GI contents, water would be pulled into the lumen resulting in an increase in water content and attendant diarrhea. In addition, with water being transported from the plasma to the chyme when hyperosmotic solutions are present in the lumen, intravascular fluid depletion would occur possibly causing hypoperfusion of tissues and organs as well as hypotension. Conversely, in the case of hypotonic GI contents, water would tend to migrate from the lumen into the interstitium thus impeding effective absorption of nutrients. The consequences of the GI tract not maintaining the luminal contents isotonic would be disastrous for whole body homeostasis.

Food molecules of various tonicities travel from the stomach to the small intestine. The GI tract amazingly maintains the isotonicity of the luminal contents, and extracellular and intravascular fluids. Isotonicity is achieved by the special functions performed by different portions of the digestive tract. The stomach secretes HCl but only absorbs a relatively small amount of it. Most absorption of fluids and food stuffs takes place in the small intestine. Small amounts of water are absorbed in the stomach. Both ethanol and aspirin are actually absorbed in the stomach because they are sufficiently water and lipid soluble in this environment to passively diffuse down a concentration gradient and across the gastric mucosa. The colon is involved in the absorption of salt and water. In addition, short chain fatty acids produced by bacteria can be passively absorbed across the colonic mucosa.

The *enterogastric reflex* regulates gastric emptying to ensure that large hypertonic loads are not continuously expelled into the duodenum since this would draw water across the relatively leaky small intestinal mucosa into the gut lumen from the circulation. As the chyme migrates into the first portion of the duodenum, H^+ ions are absorbed in exchange for Na^+ ions. In addition, iron is selectively absorbed in the duodenum. The pancreas and Brunner's glands secrete sodium bicarbonate to neutralize the gastric HCl.

Reality check 2-8: Patients with lactose intolerance lack the small intestinal brush border enzyme lactase, which breaks down lactose (milk sugar) into glucose and galactose that are smaller and are absorbed by enterocytes that prevent them from exerting osmotic effects in the lumen. Why do lactose intolerant patients present with diarrhea?

The chyme that reaches the jejunum may contain polysaccharides, triglycerides, and polypeptides, which are quickly digested to smaller molecules that are frequently osmotically active. To maintain isotonicity, special jejunal mechanisms permit the simultaneous absorption of water, electrolytes, and nutrients. If there is an inefficient absorption of water from the gut lumen, then diarrhea will occur. In contrast, excessive absorption of water across the gut lumen will result in constipation. The ileum and colon share the ability to absorb both water and electrolytes actively against big concentration gradients. The ileum is the main site for the absorption of vitamin B12 and bile salts secreted into the intestinal lumen. More details concerning sites and mechanisms of absorption and digestion may be found in other chapters of this book and other texts.

2.4.3 Gut Activity and Metabolic Factors Effect upon Intestinal Blood Flow

The splanchnic circulation includes the blood flow through the gut plus the spleen, pancreas, and liver. Under normal resting conditions, the splanchnic vasculature receives 20 % of the cardiac output and up to 40 % after a meal. During the absorption of a meal, the increase in blood flow is localized to the most active areas. Within the GI tract, blood flow is regulated lengthwise along the canal (segmental control) and between the different gut wall layers (transmural control). Both segmental and transmural controls are determined by tissue activity. Increased blood flow during increased GI activity is probably due to a combination of many factors. During digestion, several vasodilators (CCK, VIP, gastrin, and secretin) are released from the intestinal mucosa. These peptide hormones also have controlling influences on certain secretory and motor activities in the gut. Some GI glands release kallidin and bradykinin, two kinins. These kinins are very potent vasodilators and cause most of the mucosal vasodilatation that accompanies secretion. Decreased oxygen tension in the gut wall can lead to a fourfold rise in adenosine, a powerful vasodilator which could account for much of the increased blood flow.

2.4.4 Role of Immune System Cells

Immune system cells are found near the microcirculatory vessels of the GI organs. Inflammatory stimuli cause mast cells to gather around vessel smooth muscle walls and then degranulate, consequently releasing the vasoactive paracrine agents (serotonin and histamine). Prostaglandins, cytokines, leukotrienes are released by other immunologic cells.

2.4.5 Parasympathetic and Sympathetic Control of GI Blood Flow

Parasympathetic nerve stimulation to the stomach and lower colon increases local blood flow simultaneously with increased glandular secretion. The increased blood flow occurs secondary to the increased glandular secretion. Sympathetic stimulation directly decreases blood flow to the splanchnic vasculature due to intense vasoconstriction of the arterioles.

2.4.6   Countercurrent Blood Flow in the Intestinal Villus

The arterial and venous flows in intestinal villi are in opposite directions and the arterioles and venules are in close apposition. When blood initially flows into a villus, oxygen concentration is high in the arterioles but low in the venules. Hence, much of the oxygen diffuses from the arterioles to the venules (down a concentration gradient) without being carried in the blood to the villi tips. Therefore, the arterial blood oxygen content falls as the blood approaches the villus tip. Normally, this shunting of oxygen from arterioles to venules in the villi does not present a problem. However, in instances of severe reduction of blood flow to the gut, this countercurrent loss of oxygen directly contributes to the susceptibility to ischemic death of the villus. In response to ischemic injury, the intestinal villi may disintegrate and become blunted with significant decreases in intestinal absorption.

Case in Point 2-1

Chief Complaint: Diarrhea.

History: A 25-year-old man presents with fatigue and is found to have iron deficiency anemia. He has experienced episodes of intermittent mild diarrhea for many years, previously diagnosed as irritable bowel syndrome and lactose intolerance. He has no current significant gastrointestinal symptoms.

Physical Exam: Pallor and several oral aphthous ulcers. Abdominal examination is normal. The rest of the exam is unremarkable.

Labs:

Hematocrit 28 % (normal: 41–50 %), decreased mean corpuscular volume.

Leukocytes (white blood cells) $8 \times 10^3 \ \mu L^{-1}$ (normal: $3.8–10.8 \times 10^3$).

Chemistry panel and liver function tests/amylase and lipase are normal.

Stool guaiac negative for occult blood.

Recent esophagogastroduodenoscopy and colonoscopy—remarkable for celiac disease (condition in which patients have abnormal small intestinal mucosa that reverts to normal when treated with a gluten-free diet and relapse when gluten is reintroduced).

Assessment: On the basis of these findings, why does this patient experience diarrhea, bloating, and abdominal discomfort after consuming a peanut butter sandwich on whole wheat bread?

2.4.7 Recall Points

Requirements of GI Nutrient Exchange

- Most absorption takes place in the small intestine.
- Absorption occurs via active transport, diffusion, and solvent drag.
- GI tract works to maintain isotonicity of luminal contents and extracellular and intracellular fluids.

2.5 Summary Points

- The structural anatomy of the digestive system is very closely related to the physiological requirements of nutrient exchange and GI regulation.
- Signals via various receptors in the digestive system help to modulate control of motility, digestion, and absorption.
- The smooth muscle of the GI tract being unitary smooth muscle has a high degree of electrochemical coupling due to many gap junctions. Hence, the sheets or layers of smooth muscle cells contract simultaneously and act as a syncytium.
- The unitary smooth muscle exhibits characteristic slow waves or pacemaker activity.
- The characteristic pattern of slow waves determines the pattern of action potentials, which in turn establishes the frequency of contraction of the unitary smooth muscle in an organ.
- The brain–gut axis includes both an automatic and voluntary element. The digestive system can function without conscious control, by virtually having a brain of its own (ENS). Function of the digestive system can be modified by the extrinsic nervous system (parasympathetic and sympathetic nervous systems) and by GI hormones and peptides.
- Parasympathetic innervation promotes digestion and absorption by stimulating GI motility and secretions.
- Sympathetic innervation slows digestive processes by decreasing motility and secretions.
- The ENS, located in the wall of the GI tract from the esophagus to anus, consists of the myenteric plexus and the submucosal plexus.
- The myenteric or Auerbach's plexus primarily controls gut motor activity.
- The submucosal or Meissner's plexus controls secretion and blood flow within the inner wall of the gut.
- The GI peptides (e.g., hormones, paracrine agents, and neurotransmitters) regulate functions in the GI tract.
- Hormones secreted by GI enteroendocrine cells ultimately enter the systemic circulation for delivery to their target cells.
- Paracrines, released from GI tract endocrine cells, diffuse a short distance in the interstitial fluid to affect neighboring target cells.

- Neurocrines, synthesized in GI neurons, act as neurotransmitters.
- The splanchnic circulation includes blood flow through the gut, spleen, pancreas, and liver and receives between 20 and 40 % of the cardiac output.
- Most absorption of nutrients occurs in the small intestine. The colon absorbs salt and water. In addition, short chain fatty acids produced by bacteria can be passively absorbed across the colonic mucosa. Small amounts of water are absorbed in the stomach.
- Absorption through the GI mucosa occurs primarily via active transport, diffusion, and solvent drag.
- The majority of nonfat, water soluble nutrients are absorbed from the GI tract via the portal vein and temporally stored in the liver.
- The majority of fat-based nutrients are absorbed into the intestinal lymphatics and then directed to the circulating blood by the thoracic duct, bypassing the liver.
- During the absorption of a meal, increased blood flow localizes to the most active areas.
- During vigorous exercise, the arterioles of the GI tract experience intense vasoconstriction and decreased blood flow as a result of sympathetic stimulation.

2.6 Review Questions

2-1. A 30-year-old dental hygienist has been diagnosed with Scleroderma, an infiltrative connective tissue disorder that leads to increased fibrosis of the esophageal wall and LES incompetence. An esophageal motility study is performed. Which of the following conditions will she exhibit?

A. Decreased heartburn symptoms by assuming a supine position
B. Heartburn symptoms untreatable with medication
C. More efficiently clear refluxed gastric acid
D. Reduced heartburn symptoms by remaining upright for at least 2 h after a meal

2-2. A 75-year-old man is taking an anticholinergic medication called benztropine mesylate (Cogentin) for Parkinson's disease. Which of the following will this patient experience?

A. Constipation due to decreased gut motility
B. Diarrhea due to decreased gut motility
C. Diarrhea due to increased gut motility
D. No change in his gut motility

2-3. A 55-year-old patient with Zollinger–Ellison syndrome (ZES) presents to the emergency department complaining of abdominal pain and diarrhea. ZES is a disorder of gastric acid hypersecretion and severe peptic ulcer diathesis due to markedly elevated levels of gastrin from a non-beta-cell endocrine neoplasm.

Which of the following will happen to his gastric mucosal lining and acid production as a consequence of this syndrome?

A. Mucosal lining and acid production will remain the same
B. Mucosal lining will atrophy with decreased acid production
C. Mucosal lining will atrophy with increased acid production
D. Mucosal lining will increase in thickness with increased acid production

2-4. A Marine on foot patrol in Iraq has just been informed that an improvised explosive device (IED) is about to explode. As he runs for cover, which of the following changes would you expect to occur in his gastrointestinal blood flow?

A. Vasoconstriction of the splanchnic arterioles with redirection of the blood flow toward the somatic muscles
B. Vasoconstriction of the splanchnic arterioles with redirection of the blood flow toward the gut
C. Vasodilatation of his somatic arteries with redirection of blood flow toward the gut
D. Vasodilatation of the splanchnic arterioles with blood flow toward the gut

2-5. An 89-year-old woman with severe congestive heart failure complains of dull, aching chest pains when she consumes a large meal. Which of the mechanisms is the most likely cause of her ischemic chest pain?

A. Vasoconstriction of the splanchnic arterioles with the blood flow directed toward the heart
B. Vasoconstriction of the splanchnic arterioles with the blood flow directed toward the gut
C. Vasodilatation of the coronary arteries with blood directed away from the gut
D. Vasodilatation of the splanchnic arterioles with blood directed away from the coronary circulation toward the gut

2.7   Answer to Case in Point

Case in Point 2-1: To address this question first consider how the structure of the digestive system is affected by the patient's celiac disease. Ingestion of gluten in celiac disease patients leads to the production of autoantibodies and T lymphocytes to produce cytokines that damage enterocytes. Hence, exposure to gluten, the cereal protein to which the patient's small intestinal mucosa was sensitive, led to decreased absorption of fluids and nutrients due to atrophy of the mucosal lining and decreased absorptive surface area and its effects on other nutrient exchange mechanisms. Excessive amounts of unabsorbed fluids would have contributed to the patient's bouts of diarrhea. In addition, a large loss of fluids and nutrients would have also resulted in decreased weight and energy. Diminished absorption of duodenal iron would lead to iron deficiency anemia and fatigue. Mucosal atrophy and interference with the absorption of bile salts in the terminal ileum would result in fat malabsorption. Another mechanism contributing to the patient's diarrhea would be the effect of unabsorbed bile salts entering the colon when the relevant transporters are lost along the epithelium of the terminal ileum. In addition, effacement of the terminal ileal mucosa would contribute to vitamin B12 deficiency and an erythrocyte deficiency, pernicious anemia. By adhering to a gluten-free diet, the patient's intestinal mucosa was allowed to return to a more normal state. Hence, effective and efficient fluid and nutrient exchange was reestablished.

2.8   Answer to Connecting-the-Dots

Connecting-the-Dots 2-1: The patient's loss of peripheral reflexes coupled with decreased intestinal motility is indicative of hypokalemia. Indeed the patient's serum potassium measured at the time of the chloride measurement was just 2.3 mmol/L (normal 3.5–5). Potassium diminished, like the chloride, because of the large loss of gastric secretion. The decline in blood potassium, and hence in extracellular spaces of muscle, alters the potassium electrochemical gradient that is essential for normal nerve function. The role of potassium is to repolarize the cell membrane to its resting state after the action potential has passed. The hypokalemia leads to hyperpolarization of the resting membrane potential thus requiring a greater than normal stimulus to initiate a new action potential. This increased demand leads to loss of reflexes and can even cause paralysis. Administration of potassium chloride to the patient allowed the cecostomy to begin functioning and muscle function also returned to normal.

2.9   Answers to Reality Checks

Reality check 2-1: Sjögren's syndrome is a chronic autoimmune disease in which white blood cells attack their moisture-producing glands. Today, as many as four million Americans live with this disease. We would expect the tennis superstar to experience a dry mouth and decreased lubricating secretions in the GI tract. In addition, she would probably show a decreased ability to produce tears in the face of an emotional victory.

   Reality check 2-2: Patients with scleroderma involving the esophagus experience difficulty swallowing solids and liquids due to hardening of the connective tissues. This scenario greatly compromises esophageal peristalsis and the propulsion of boluses toward the stomach. In addition, due to fibrotic infiltration of the LES, patients also experience gastroesophageal reflux.

Reality check 2-3: Hirschsprung's disease results from a lack of ganglion cells of the involved colonic segment. In this case, the aganglionic sigmoid colon does not relax and causes an obstruction. One would expect dilation of the colon above the level of the sigmoid colon.

Reality check 2-4: The superior mesenteric artery supplies blood to the right and part of the transverse colon. These would be the areas under consideration for colonic resection.

Reality check 2-5: Parasympathetic innervation to the gastrointestinal tract is supplied by the vagus and pelvic nerves. The parasympathetic postganglionic neurons are classified as cholinergic or peptidergic. ACh is the neurotransmitter released from cholinergic neurons which lead to an increase in GI motility and secretions. Atropine is an anticholinergic agent. Therefore, you would expect a patient receiving atropine to experience a decrease in peristalsis and secretions.

Reality check 2-6: Complete transection of the spinal cord at the C4 level would cause a major alteration in the brain–gut axis. Spinal cord injury damages nerves that allow a patient to control bowel movements. Above the T-12 level, the patient may lose the ability to feel when the rectum is full and requires emptying. In addition, the anal sphincter remains tight. In these patients, when the rectum is full a defecation reflex occurs and the bowel empties. Hence, patients with spinal cord injuries above T-12 lose volitional bowel control and suffer from constipation. In contrast, patients with a spinal cord injury below the T-12 level experience a weakened defecation reflex and decreased anal sphincter strength. This results in a flaccid bowel and incontinence.

Reality check 2-7: CCK injection leads to gallbladder contraction, sphincter of Oddi relaxation, and the secretion of bile into the duodenal lumen. When the endoscopists see the bile enter the duodenum that alerts them to search in that area for the ampulla which communicates with the bile duct.

Reality check 2-8: Patients with lactose intolerance lack the lactase brush border enzyme. Therefore, the lactose cannot be broken down to the smaller molecules of glucose and galactose which are absorbed by enterocytes. Their normal absorption prevents them from exerting osmotic effects in the lumen. When lactose cannot be absorbed in its parent form, it presents a large osmotic load that draws water into the gut lumen if it is not broken down by the enzyme lactase.

2.10 Answers to Review Questions

2-1. **D**. Scleroderma is an infiltrative connective tissue disorder, which in this case results in decreased esophageal peristalsis and an incompetent LES. These combined defects will lead to gastroesophageal reflux of stomach acid. In general, when a patient waits for 2 h after consuming a meal, the gastric contents should empty to some degree. Therefore, a smaller volume of gastric contents versus none would be available for reflux. In addition, the clearance of the refluxate will be aided by gravity when the patient is upright.

2-2. **A.** Benztropine mesylate (Cogentin) is an anticholinergic medication. In general, cholinergic innervation leads to increased gut motility. Therefore, when given an anticholinergic medication, the patient should experience decreased gut motility and constipation.

2-3. **D.** ZES is a disorder of gastric acid hypersecretion and severe peptic ulcer diathesis due to hypersecretion of gastrin from non-beta-cell endocrine neoplasm. Gastrin secretion results in increased stomach acid production, increased thickness of the stomach mucosal lining, and increased stomach motility. Thus, in a ZES patient with hypergastrinemia, one would expect both stomach acid secretion and stomach mucosal lining to be increased.

2-4. **A.** The vigorous exercise induced by running away from an explosive device results in sympathetic nervous stimulation to the gut. The GI tract arterioles experience intense vasoconstriction and decreased blood flow which would direct blood flow away from the gut and toward the somatic muscles to aid in flight.

2-5. **D.** During the absorption of a meal, the increase in blood flow is localized to the most active areas in the gut. When this elderly patient consumes a large meal, blood is shifted away from her systemic circulation toward her splanchnic circulation. In a patient with a poor cardiac pump, even a relatively small diversion of blood flow would result in lower blood flow to the heart and ischemic cardiac pain.

Suggested Reading

Costanzo LS. Physiology. 4th ed. Philadelphia: Saunders; 2010. Chapter 8, Gastrointestinal Physiology; p. 327–78.

Fenoglio-Preiser CM, Noffsinger AE, Stemmermann GN, Lantz PE, Isaacson PG. Gastrointestinal physiology. 3rd ed. Philadelphia: Lippincott Williams & Wilkins; 2008. Chapter 1, General features of the gastrointestinal tract and evaluation of specimens derived from it; p. 1–10.

Janson LW, Tischler ME. The big picture: medical biochemistry. New York: McGraw Hill; 2012. Chapter 11, The digestive system; p. 149–66.

Chapter 3
Brain–Gut Axis and Regional Gastrointestinal Tract Motility

3.1 Introduction

The GI tract works "around the clock" to supply the body with nutrients for energy, growth, and repair. Over 24 h, the GI tract facilitates the delivery on average of 1,850–2,550 cal from foodstuffs coupled with the absorption of 2 L of dietary liquids and 7 L of combined salivary, gastric, pancreaticobiliary, and intestinal secretions. This process requires the coordination of chewing, swallowing, and gastrointestinal motility to support digestion and absorption. The brain–gut axis (i.e., the central nervous system [CNS], enteric nervous system [ENS], and the enteroendocrine cells) serves as the coordinating system that controls GI motor functions. Some questions arise relevant to GI motility. What determines the size of food particles for absorption in the small intestine? What role do gut motor functions play in the rate of absorption of food particles and fluids? What factors determine fecal excretion? Gastrointestinal motility plays a pivotal role in supporting nutrient processing and transportation. Each region of the GI tract has its own unique contribution to make in the process.

3.2 Food Ingestion and Deglutition

3.2.1 Mechanics of Mastication

Mastication (chewing) includes both involuntary and voluntary components. Initiation of reflexes begins with placement of food in the mouth. Oral mechanoreceptors relay sensory information to the brain stem, which coordinates a pattern of muscle activity that results in chewing due to alternating contraction and relaxation of the jaw muscles. Nuclei in the brain stem control the process of mastication, and the motor (mandibular) branch of the fifth cranial nerve (trigeminal nerve) innervates the majority of muscles of mastication (Fig. 3.1).

E. Trowers and M. Tischler, *Gastrointestinal Physiology*, 37
DOI 10.1007/978-3-319-07164-0_3, © Springer International Publishing Switzerland 2014

Fig. 3.1 Innervation of muscles used in chewing. Fifth cranial nerve showing its motor root innervates the majority of muscles of mastication via the mandibular branch

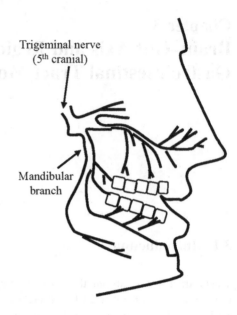

Trigeminal nerve
(5th cranial)

Mandibular
branch

3.2.2 Main Functions of Mastication

There are three main functions of mastication. First, chewing breaks down food boluses into smaller particles to facilitate the act of swallowing. Second, during chewing, food mixes with saliva. This process of lubrication of the food particles also makes swallowing easier. Finally, salivary amylase mixing with ingested carbohydrates initiates their digestion.

Reality check 3-1: An elderly woman has undergone extensive head and neck radiation therapy due to malignant lymphoma involving her salivary glands bilaterally. What would happen to her ability to lubricate food particles? What would happen to her ability to initiate carbohydrate digestion?

3.2.3 Deglutition

Stages of Deglutition: *Deglutition*, the medical term for swallowing, involves three stages: (1) a voluntary stage, (2) a pharyngeal stage, which is predominantly involuntary and is responsible for transporting the food bolus from the pharynx into the esophagus, and (3) an esophageal stage, which is involuntary and is responsible for transporting the food bolus from the pharynx into the stomach (Fig. 3.2).

Takeru Kobayashi holds several records, including four Guinness Records, for eating hot dogs, meatballs, Twinkies, hamburgers, and pasta. The 131 lb wonder is truly one of the fastest eaters on the planet. He expands his stomach for a

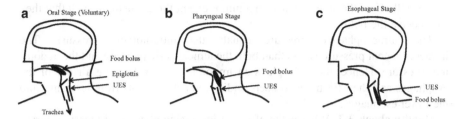

Fig. 3.2 The three stages of swallowing. (**a**) The voluntary stage in which the food bolus is in the mouth and the epiglottis has not yet blocked the tracheal opening. (**b**) The pharyngeal stage which is predominantly involuntary and is responsible for transporting the food bolus from the pharynx into the esophagus with the epiglottis blocking the opening to the trachea. (**c**) The esophageal stage which is involuntary and is responsible for transporting the food bolus from the pharynx into the stomach. *UES* upper esophageal sphincter

competition by eating larger and larger amounts of food, and then exercises to ensure that fat will not impede expansion of his stomach during a competition. He uses a trademark body wiggle to force food down his esophagus and settle more compactly in his stomach.

As a food bolus enters the mouth the tongue voluntarily forces the bolus back toward the pharynx, which has a high concentration of somatosensory receptors. The activation of the somatosensory receptors triggers the involuntary deglutition reflex in the medulla. The soft palate is pulled upward and closes the posterior nares. This action prevents food from being refluxed into the nasal cavities. The epiglottis covers the laryngeal opening and the larynx moves upward against the epiglottis to keep food from entering the trachea. The upper esophageal sphincter (UES) relaxes which allows the food bolus to travel from the pharynx to the esophagus. The initiation of a peristaltic wave in the pharynx moves the bolus through the open UES. Respiration is inhibited during the pharyngeal stage of swallowing.

As the food bolus exits the pharynx, the swallowing reflex coordinates the opening of the UES, which allows the bolus to enter the esophagus. The UES closes when the bolus is in the esophagus. Closure of the UES at this time prevents reflux of the bolus into the pharynx. Two types of peristaltic waves occur in the esophagus: (1) primary peristalsis, which is mediated by the swallowing reflex and begun in the pharynx, and (2) secondary peristalsis. A primary peristaltic wave is a coordinated sequence of contractions in which, as each segment of the esophagus contracts, a region of high pressure immediately behind the bolus propels it down the esophagus (see Fig. 2.3). If the bolus is not cleared from the esophagus, then a secondary peristaltic wave arises due to the distention of the esophageal wall. The ENS mediates the secondary peristaltic wave, which continues until all of the bolus is cleared from the esophagus.

As the bolus approaches the lower esophagus, the lower esophageal sphincter (LES) opens due to the action of myenteric inhibitory neurons that release VIP as its neurotransmitter. In addition, the wave of relaxation that precedes the peristaltic waves will affect the stomach, and to a minor extent the duodenum, such that they can receive the bolus.

The intraesophageal pressure equals the intrathoracic pressure. The intraesophageal pressure is less than both the atmospheric pressure and the abdominal pressure. Hence, the UES plays an important role in keeping air out of the esophagus and the LES helps to keep acidic stomach contents from refluxing into the lower esophagus.

Reality check 3-2: What is the effect of increasing abdominal pressure during pregnancy on the LES? How can this contribute to increasing heartburn symptoms as the pregnancy progresses?

3.2.4   Recall Points

Food Ingestion and Deglutition
• Mastication (involuntary/voluntary)
• Deglutition (involuntary/voluntary)

3.3   Gastric Motor Functions

The stomach anatomy includes several defined regions (Fig. 3.3a). The *cardia* is located near the gastroesophageal junction. The *fundus* is the rounded portion of the stomach located above the gastroesophageal sphincter. The *body* or *corpus* comprises the primary volume of the stomach. The lower part of the stomach, the *pylorus*, connecting the stomach to the duodenum includes the *pyloric antrum*, the initial part that connects to the body, and the *pyloric canal*, which connects to the duodenum separated by the *pyloric spincter*. The *orad* portion of the stomach includes the fundus plus proximal or upper body. The *caudad* portion of the stomach includes the antrum and distal or lower body.

There are three motor functions associated with the stomach. First, the *orad* region relaxes to allow a food bolus to move from the esophagus into the stomach (Fig. 3.3b). This receptive relaxation is triggered by the food bolus causing distention in the lower esophagus and is a *vagovagal reflex* which is abolished by *vagotomy* (vagus nerve resection). As the associated peristaltic contraction moves toward the stomach, it initiates a preceding wave of relaxation due to myenteric neurons which release VIP acting as an inhibitory transmitter. This wave of relaxation causes the stomach, and to a lesser degree the duodenum, to relax and receive the food bolus from the esophagus. During receptive relaxation gastric pressure decreases and gastric volume increases.

Second, stomach contractions, which decrease the size of the food bolus and mix it with gastric secretions, result in the production of the semifluid mixture called chyme. The *caudad* includes a thick muscular wall, which produces the

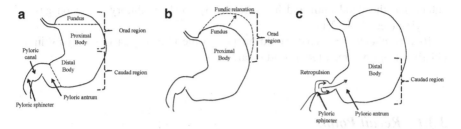

Fig. 3.3 Gastric motor functions. (**a**) The fundus, body, and antrum are the major divisions of the stomach. The orad region includes fundus and upper body and the caudad region the antrum and lower body. (**b**) The fundus relaxes (*dotted line*) to accommodate the food bolus. The antrum then grinds the food and pumps the chime into the duodenum through the pyloric sphincter. (**c**) Gastric retropulsion further mixes and reduces food particle size

contractions needed for mixing, propulsion, and the reduction of the size of food particles. The slow wave *basic electrical rhythm* (BER), or gastric pacemaker, occurs in the wall of the caudad stomach at a rate of 3–5 waves/min and depolarize the gastric smooth muscle cells. As these gastric contractions move downward from the caudad region of the stomach toward the antrum, they increase in intensity. These waves of contraction result in the mixing of the gastric contents and propel some of the chyme from the pylorus into the duodenum. The wave of contraction also results in the closure of the pylorus. Closure of the pylorus forces the majority of the gastric contents back into the stomach for more mixing and reduction of food particle size via the process called *retropulsion* (Fig. 3.3c). Vagal stimulation, gastrin release, and local distention increase gastric contractions. Sympathetic stimulation as well as the hormones secretin and Gastric inhibitory peptide (GIP) results in a decrease in the force of gastric contractions.

Third, slow emptying of chyme from the stomach into the duodenum allows for the appropriate amount of time for digestion and absorption of nutrients in the small bowel. The normal gastric food volume after a meal is ~1.5 L. The time it takes for the gastric contents to travel to the duodenum is about 2–3 h. The relative speed of gastric emptying for food substances from fastest to slowest is liquids → carbohydrates → proteins → fats. Gastric emptying is controlled to a lesser extent by gastric causes, e.g., distention of the stomach wall or the *promotility* effect of gastrin on gastric peristalsis. Potent duodenal factors play the major role in suppressing gastric emptying by eliciting *enterogastric reflexes*. Examples of the potent duodenal factors that suppress gastric emptying include significant distention of the duodenal wall, the low pH (acidity) of chyme in the duodenum, hyper- or hypotonicity of the chyme, and the increased amount of fats and certain protein breakdown products. The presence of fats in the duodenum triggers the release of the hormone cholecystokinin (CCK), which competitively inhibits gastrin's promotility effect on the stomach (see Table 2.1). GIP, a hormone, is secreted by the upper small intestine primarily in response to the presence of fat and to a lesser extent carbohydrates in the duodenal chyme (see Table 2.1). The hormone secretin is released from the duodenal mucosal lining in response to gastric acid, which enters into the duodenum and has a relatively weak inhibitory effect on gastric emptying (see Table 2.1).

Reality check 3-3: What would happen to the rate of gastric emptying in an elderly edentulous man fed a solid meal?

3.3.1 Recall Points

Gastric Motor Functions
- Components of gastric motility.
- Stimulation of gastric motility.
- Roles of parasympathetic innervation, gastrin, and local distention.
- Inhibition of gastric motility via acidic contents and the inhibition of gastrin release.
- Duodenal, neural, and hormonal feedback.

Case in Point 3-1

Chief Complaint: Crampy abdominal pain and diarrhea.

History: A 69-year-old man returns to your clinic for follow-up of chronic abdominal pain. He is well known to clinic staff, as he has a past history of a perforated peptic ulcer for which he had a truncal vagotomy. Today he states that he occasionally experiences burning midepigastric pain which is alleviated by over-the-counter antacids. He states that 30–60 min after consuming a can of a hyperosmolar nutrient supplement, he experiences diarrhea, bloating, and crampy abdominal pain. His review of systems and past medical history are otherwise unremarkable.

Physical Exam: An elderly man in no acute distress. Vital signs are temperature 98.6 °F, blood pressure 120/82 mmHg, pulse 78 per minute, and respirations 14 per minute. Physical examination of the skin reveals a well-healed abdominal surgical scar and is otherwise normal.

Labs:

Hematocrit 44 % (normal: 41–50 %).

Leukocytes (white blood cells) 8×10^3 μL^{-1} (normal: $3.8–10.8 \times 10^3$).

Mean corpuscular volume/chemistry panel and liver function tests/amylase and lipase are normal.

Stool guaiac negative for occult blood.

Results of recent esophagogastroduodenoscopy and colonoscopy are unremarkable.

Assessment: On the basis of these findings, why does this patient experience diarrhea, bloating, and abdominal discomfort after consuming a hyperosmolar nutrient supplement?

3.4   Small Bowel Motor Functions

The small intestines function primarily concerns the digestion and absorption of nutrients. The small intestine mixes the chyme with digestive enzymes via segmentation contractions initiated by distention of the small bowel wall by chyme. The resultant small bowel distention triggers regularly spaced concentric contractions along the length of the small intestine causing segmentations that last for less than a minute (see Fig. 2.7). The frequency of the slow waves or BER in the small bowel (12 waves/min) sets the frequency of the segmentation. Mixing takes place when a segment of the small bowel contracts and splits the chyme into an orad and caudad portion. When that segment of small bowel relaxes, the orad and caudad portions of the chyme intermix without any effective forward movement of the chyme. Small bowel peristaltic contractions move chyme through the small intestine in the direction of the anus. Contraction of the small bowel wall behind (orad) the chyme couples with the relaxation in front of (caudad) the chyme which results in the propelling of the chyme in the analward or caudad direction. Acetylcholine and Substance P, neurotransmitters, trigger the orad component of small bowel peristaltic contractions, whereas VIP and nitric oxide play this role for the caudad relaxation component. Small bowel peristalsis largely increases after a meal due to the gastroenteric reflex triggered by gastric wall distention and transmitted from the stomach wall downward along the small intestinal wall via the myenteric plexus. In addition, several hormones increase small bowel peristalsis, e.g., thyroid hormone, gastrin, CCK, and insulin (Fig. 3.4). On the other hand, secretin and glucagon decrease small bowel peristalsis. Primarily the ileocecal sphincter prevents the backflow of colonic contents into the small intestine (Fig. 3.5). Increased cecal pressure or chemical irritation in the cecum will decrease peristalsis in the ileum and increase contraction of the ileocecal sphincter. On the other hand, increased pressure and chemical irritation in the ileum will result in relaxation of the ileocecal sphincter and increased peristalsis.

Reality check 3-4: A college student has been shot at point blank range. He has sustained major trauma to his small intestines which will need a 60–70 % small bowel resection. You are the house officer talking with the patient's parents while the patient is being rushed into the operating suite. The parents want to know what happens when an individual is left with a relatively short segment of small bowel?

3.4.1   Recall Points

Small Bowel Motor Functions
- Mixing (segmentation) and propulsive (peristaltic) contractions.
- Relaxation of ileosphincter due to ileal distention.
- Contraction of ileosphincter due to colonic distention.

Fig. 3.4 Hormones that affect small bowel peristalsis

Hormones increasing peristalsis:
CCK
Gastrin
Insulin
Thyroid hormone

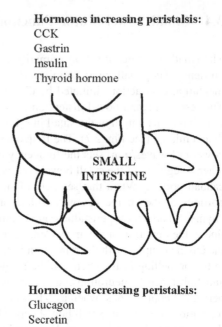

Hormones decreasing peristalsis:
Glucagon
Secretin

3.5   Large Bowel Motor Functions

The absorption of water and electrolytes from chyme, which produces feces (proximal colon) and the storage of feces (distal colon), serves as the main roles of the large intestine (Fig. 3.5). Segmentation contractions occur in a similar fashion to those in the small intestine and produce saclike segments in the proximal colon called haustra. These colonic segmentation contractions serve to mix the large bowel contents as well as facilitate the exposure of the fecal material to the large bowel mucosal surface with resultant absorption of fluid and dissolved substances. Mass movements propel the large bowel contents over long distances, e.g., from the beginning of the transverse colon to the sigmoid colon. These mass movements occur between one and three times per day and are a derivative form of peristalsis. Mass movements may be triggered after a meal due to gastrocolic (distention of the stomach) or gastroduodenal (distention of the duodenum) reflexes. In addition, colonic irritation may also precipitate mass movements.

Defecation involves both involuntary (reflex) and voluntary activities. In general the rectum is devoid of feces. The *rectosphincteric reflex* causes the rectum to contract and the internal anal sphincter to relax when the rectum begins to fill with feces. When the rectum becomes 25 % filled one develops an urge to have a bowel movement. However, this urge to defecate is thwarted by the tonically contracted external anal sphincter. When it is opportune to defecate, the external anal sphincter is voluntarily relaxed and the rectal smooth muscle contracts, propelling the feces from the anorectum. By expiring against a closed glottis (*Valsalva maneuver*), one can increase the intra-abdominal pressure for defecation.

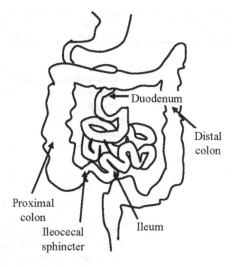

Fig. 3.5 Anatomical relationship of small and large intestine. The ileocecal sphincter prevents the backflow of colonic contents into the small intestine (ileal portion). Increased cecal pressure or chemical irritation in the cecum will increase contraction of the ileocecal sphincter. On the other hand, increased pressure and chemical irritation in the ileum will result in relaxation of the ileocecal sphincter. The main roles of the large intestine are the absorption of water and electrolytes from chyme to produce feces (proximal colon) and store feces (distal colon). Colonic segmentation contractions mix the large bowel contents as well as facilitate exposure of the fecal material to the large bowel mucosal surface with resultant absorption of fluid and dissolved substances

The key regional GI motor functions and their brain–gut axis regulation are summarized in Table 3.1.

Connecting-the-Dots 3-1

You are a fourth year medical student on a GI elective rotation. This week you are in the GI clinic. Eager to make a good impression on your GI attending, you eagerly volunteer to see the patient in room 3 who was referred by her primary care physician for an evaluation of chronic diarrhea (greater than 6–8 weeks duration). Upon conducting a focused history, physical exam, and assessment of the patient's labs and special labs, you note that the patient complains of diaphoresis (sweating), 25 lb weight loss, heat intolerance, and irritability. Physical examination reveals a slender 20-year-old woman with exophthalmos (prominent eyes due to an infiltrative opthalmopathy) and a prominent goiter. Her laboratory studies reveal a suppressed TSH and increased T_4, FT_4, T_3, and FT_3. You left your PDA in your car, but you go online and search a reputable medical search engine and determine that your patient has hyperthyroidism due to Graves' disease, which is the most common cause of thyrotoxicosis. What links can you make between accelerated regional GI tract motility and the patient's GI symptoms in your analysis of this case?

Table 3.1 Regional GI motor functions and their brain–gut axis regulation

GI motor function and location	Brain axis/neural regulation
Mouth	
Mastication (chewing)	• Voluntary control: brain stem nuclei regulate jaw muscle contraction/relaxation by activating the trigeminal nerve (cranial nerve V) leading to the mandibular branch
	• Involuntary control: oral mechanoreceptors and muscle stretch receptors signal the central pattern generator of the CNS
Esophagus	
Deglutition (swallowing)	• Tongue forces bolus toward the pharynx (voluntary)
• Voluntary stage	• Pharyngeal somatosensory receptors trigger involuntary deglutition reflex in medulla (CNS) via afferent impulses (pharyngeal)
• Pharyngeal stage	• Pharyngeal branches of superior laryngeal branch of vagus to medulla coordinates pharyngeal spasm and initiation of esophageal peristalsis
• Esophageal stage	• ENS mediated secondary peristaltic wave (esophageal)
Stomach	
• Receptive relaxation: food bolus leaves esophagus	• Vagovagal reflex due to distention of lower esophagus relaxes orad region to accept food bolus from esophagus (receptive relaxation)
• Muscle contractions: decrease bolus size; mix with secretions to produce chyme	• Vagal stimulation increases gastric muscle contractions
• Ejection of chyme	• Primary control of gastric motility is integrative centers in the brain stem
	• ENS-mediated peristalsis of lower stomach (caudad region) helps to promote grinding
Small intestine	
• Chyme mixed with digestive enzymes	• ENS-mediated peristalsis of small intestine mixes chyme with digestive enzymes
• Chyme moved into colon	• Peristalsis moves chyme toward the anus
Large intestine	
• Colonic absorption of water/electrolytes	• ENS-mediated peristalsis of large intestine moves contents toward the anus
• Formation and storage of stool	• Colonic segmentation exposes fecal matter to mucosa for fluid absorption
• Movement of stool toward rectum	• Mass movements propel contents
• Defecation	• Feces distend rectum; stretch receptors (rectosphincteric reflex) send afferent signals to spinal cord leading to rectum contraction (pelvic nerve spinal reflex)
	• Inhibition of voluntary motor neurons relaxes external anal sphincter

Reality check 3-5: Irritable bowel syndrome (IBS) is a disorder of colonic motility in which patients may experience bouts of diarrhea, constipation, or both. Why would patients with increased segmentation contractions experience constipation? Why would patients with decreased segmentation contractions experience diarrhea?

Reality check 3-6: Patients with high grade distal colonic obstruction due to large tumors may present with diarrhea. Why?

3.5.1 Recall Points

Large Bowel Motor Functions
- Peristalsis
- Haustrations (segmentation contractions)
- Mass movements

3.6 Summary Points

- The brain–gut axis includes the CNS, ENS, and the enteroendocrine cells and is the coordinating system which controls GI motor functions.
- Mastication (chewing) includes involuntary and voluntary components. Nuclei in the brain stem control the process of mastication. The fifth cranial nerve's motor branch innervates the majority of the muscles of mastication. Mastication breaks down food into smaller pieces and mixes food particles with saliva which facilitates swallowing.
- Deglutition (swallowing) involves three stages: (1) voluntary, (2) pharyngeal that is predominantly involuntary and is responsible for transporting food from the pharynx into the esophagus, and (3) esophageal which is involuntary and responsible for transporting food from the pharynx into the stomach.
- Control of gastric emptying occurs via potent duodenal factors, e.g., distention of the duodenal wall, acidity and hyper-or hypotonicity of chyme in the duodenum, and the increased amount of fats and certain protein breakdown products.
- Vagal stimulation, gastrin release, and local distention increase gastric contractions.
- The frequency of small bowel segmentation contractions is set by the frequency of the slow waves or BER which is 12 waves/min. Segmentation results in mixing of the chyme in preparation for digestion and absorption.
- Acetylcholine and Substance P, neurotransmitters, trigger the orad component of small bowel peristaltic contractions. VIP and nitric oxide serve in the same way for the caudad relaxation component.
- Thyroid hormone, gastrin, CCK, and insulin increase small bowel peristalsis.
- Secretin and glucagon decrease small bowel peristalsis.

- The ileocecal sphincter prevents backflow of colonic contents into the small bowel.
- Ileocecal sphincter contraction increases in response to increased cecal pressure or chemical irritation in the cecum.
- Ileocecal sphincter contraction decreases in response to increased pressure and chemical irritation in the ileum.
- Haustra are colonic segmentation contractions which serve to mix the large bowel contents and facilitate the exposure of fecal material to the colonic mucosal surface for absorption of fluid and dissolved substances.
- Mass movements propel colonic contents over long distances one to three times per day.
- Defecation involves involuntary and voluntary activities. In general, the rectum is devoid of feces. When it becomes 25 % filled, one develops an urge to defecate.
- When it is opportune to have a bowel movement, the external anal sphincter relaxes and the rectal smooth muscle contracts which propels the feces from the anorectum.

3.7   Review Questions

3-1. Achalasia is an esophageal motility disorder in which patients present with absent/decreased lower esophageal wall muscular contractions due to a loss of ganglion cells and an inability of the LES to relax. In patients with achalasia, which of the following conditions is most likely to be correct?

   A. Can swallow without difficulty
   B. Require less time than an average person to propel food from their esophagus into their stomach
   C. Require more time than an average person to propel food from their esophagus into their stomach
   D. Unable to regurgitate

3-2. The BER, or gastric pacemaker, is a slow wave that occurs in the wall of the caudad stomach at a rate of 3–5 waves/min and depolarizes the gastric smooth muscle cells which sets the maximal frequency of contraction. Which of the following statements correctly describes a characteristic of the wave of gastric contractions?

   A. Is very weak and does not affect the gastric contents
   B. Results in the mixing of gastric contents
   C. Results in the segmentation of gastric contents
   D. Results in the separation of the gastric contents

3-3. A 27-year-old nursing student suffered a perforation of her appendix with abscess formation. During surgery the decision was made to resect the distal portion of her terminal ileum including her ileocecal sphincter. Which of the following problems will the patient most likely experience?

A. Constipation because the fecal stream will have more contact time for absorption
B. Constipation due to decreased gut motility
C. Diarrhea because the fecal stream will have less contact time for absorption
D. Diarrhea because the fecal stream will have more contact time for absorption

3-4. Colonoscopy is a procedure performed to diagnose and treat problems of the large intestine. Colonoscopy is conducted using a lighted flexible tube that allows the physician to see inside the colon. A 79-year-old patient with multiple diverticulae (blind pouches) has a very spastic colon making visualization of the lumen and mucosal lining difficult. Which of the following substances should the colonoscopist administer IV to decrease peristalsis and enhance visualization?

A. CCK
B. Gastrin
C. Glucagon
D. Insulin

3-5. A 28-year-old allied health student has been diagnosed with Crohn's disease, an infiltrative inflammatory bowel disorder which leads to increased fibrosis of transmural thickness of his large bowel. Which of the following problems will this patient most likely suffer?

A. Constipation due to increased absorption of water from the colon
B. Constipation due to increased colonic motility
C. Diarrhea due to decreased absorption of water from the colon
D. Diarrhea due to increased absorption of water from the colon

3.8 Answer to Case in Point

Case in Point 3-1: As a consequence of the complete vagotomy, receptive relaxation in the stomach is abolished. Hence, the stomach loses much of its reservoir capacity. The hyperosmolar nutrient supplement is not held in the stomach long enough for proper processing. Therefore, the more hyperosmolar nutrient supplement leaves the stomach and enters into the small bowel where its more osmotically active particles attract water into the gut lumen which results in bloating, crampy abdominal pain, and diarrhea.

3.9   Answer to Connecting the Dots

Connecting-the-Dots 3-1: An understanding of regional GI tract motility will help us assess this patient's chronic diarrhea. Thyroid hormone stimulates the stomach to empty faster. In addition, both small and large bowel peristalsis increases. The chyme and fecal stream consequently spend less time in contact with the mucosal lining resulting in less absorption of luminal fluid and nutrients from the intestines and subsequent diarrhea. This loss of fluid and nutrients contributes to dehydration and weight loss. Restoring the patient to a euthyroid state likewise restores her fluid and nutrient balance.

3.10   Answers to Reality Checks

Reality check 3-1: During chewing, food mixes with saliva which serves to lubricate the food particles and make swallowing easier. With extensive radiation injury to her salivary glands, this elderly woman would have difficulty swallowing her food due to decreased saliva production. In addition, carbohydrate digestion is initiated when salivary amylase mixes with ingested carbohydrates. Hence, one would expect this elderly woman to have difficulty in her ability to initiate carbohydrate digestion as well.

Reality check 3-2: During pregnancy, increasing abdominal pressure would increase pressure on the gastric side of the LES and potentiate esophageal reflux to occur. Other hormonal factors may also contribute to increasing the likelihood of esophageal reflux during pregnancy.

Reality check 3-3: Gastric emptying time might be prolonged in an elderly edentulous man to allow the stomach contractions more time to decrease the size of the larger food boluses which normally would have been broken down into smaller pieces by the teeth.

Reality check 3-4: This unfortunate student will suffer from short bowel syndrome (SBS). SBS afflicts patients who have at least half of their small bowel resected. Basically, these patients may become malnourished because they are not able to absorb sufficient nutrients, water, and vitamins. These patients risk developing dehydration, weakness, weight loss, and infections.

Reality check 3-5: Colonic segmentation contractions serve to mix the large bowel contents as well as facilitate the exposure of the fecal material to the large bowel mucosal surface with resultant absorption of fluid and dissolved substances. If a patient has increased segmentation contractions his/her fecal contents would experience enhanced contact time with the large bowel mucosal surface which would result in more absorption of fluid and constipation. If a patient has decreased segmentation contractions his/her fecal contents would experience diminished contact time with the large bowel mucosal surface which would result in less absorption of fluid and diarrhea.

Reality check 3-6: Most of the fluid is absorbed in the proximal half of the colon. Hence, stool in the left colon tends to be solid. In patients with a high grade obstruction, liquid stool can more easily pass through the obstructed segment compared to solid stool. Hence, these patients present with a postobstructive diarrhea.

3.11 Answers to Review Questions

3-1. **C.** Achalasia is an esophageal motility disorder in which patients present with absent lower esophageal wall muscular contractions due to a loss/decrease of ganglion cells and an inability of the LES to relax. These combined defects will result in poor clearance of food from the esophagus and a prolongation of the time to consume a meal. Patients with achalasia frequently experience difficulty with swallowing and may experience regurgitation.

3-2. **B.** The BER of the stomach or gastric pacemaker is a slow wave which occurs in the wall of the caudad stomach at a rate of 3–5 waves/min and depolarizes the gastric smooth muscle cells which in turn set the maximal frequency of contraction. As the gastric contractions move downward from the caudad region of the stomach toward the antrum they increase in intensity. These waves of contraction result in the mixing of the gastric contents and propel some of the chyme from the pylorus into the duodenum.

3-3. **C.** The ileocecal sphincter plays an important role in controlling the rate of the fecal stream entry into the large intestine. If the ileocecal sphincter or "ileocecal brake" is surgically removed the patient will experience diarrhea because the fecal stream will have less contact time for absorption.

3-4. **C.** The colonoscopist should consider administering IV glucagon to decrease peristalsis in the colon. This would make it easier to visualize the bowel wall and help with the maneuvering of the scope. IV glucagon can also lead to an increase in blood glucose; hence, its use should be avoided in diabetic patients.

3-5. **C.** The absorption of water and electrolytes from chyme occurs primarily in the proximal colon. If a patient has an increased transmural thickness of his/her colonic wall due to Crohn's disease then he/she will suffer from diarrhea due to decreased absorption of water.

Suggested Reading

Barrett KE, Barman SM, Boitano S, Brooks HL. Ganong's review of medical physiology. 24th ed. New York: McGraw Hill Lange; 2012. Chapter 27, Gastrointestinal motility; p. 497–508.

Hasler WL. Motility of the small intestine and colon. In: Yamada T, Alpers DH, Kalloo AN, Kaplowitz N, Owyang C, Powell DW, editors. Textbook of gastroenterology. 5th ed. Oxford: Wiley; 2009. Chapter 11.

Kahrilas PJ, Pandolfino JE. Esophageal motor function. In: Yamada T, Alpers DH, Kalloo AN, Kaplowitz N, Owyang C, Powell DW, editors. Textbook of gastroenterology. 5th ed. Oxford: Wiley; 2009. Chapter 9.

Chapter 4
Gastrointestinal Secretion: Aids in Digestion and Absorption

4.1 Introduction

Having read about characteristics of ingestion, swallowing, and other aspects of regional GI motility, we now examine the relevant anatomy and factors involved in GI secretion. In an integrated approach to GI function, it is logical to discuss gastric mucosal function after salivary secretion followed by pancreatic and biliary secretory processes because they respond to what happens during gastric digestion and emptying. Additionally, we will continue to focus on the regulatory role of the brain–gut axis in this chapter. In Chap. 3 the elements of the brain–gut axis working together to coordinate and control GI tract motility were outlined. This chapter examines the controlling factors in GI secretion and the interplay of the brain–gut axis.

4.2 Salivary Gland Secretions

4.2.1 Serous Versus Mucous

The three sets of paired salivary glands include *parotid*, *submaxillary*, and *sublingual*. Grossly, the salivary glands resemble a bunch of grapes. A single grape corresponds to an acinus, which is the blind end of a branching duct system lined by *acinar cells* (Fig. 4.1a). Serous secretion and mucus secretion are the two main types of protein secretion. Serous secretion contains ptyalin, which is an enzyme classified as an alpha amylase and is utilized in starch digestion.

E. Trowers and M. Tischler, *Gastrointestinal Physiology*,
DOI 10.1007/978-3-319-07164-0_4, © Springer International Publishing Switzerland 2014

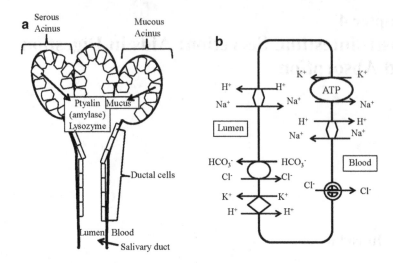

Fig. 4.1 Salivary gland. (**a**) Structure of the salivary gland with serous and mucus cell secretions. (**b**) Salivary duct ion transporters. ATP = Na–K ATPase pump

4.2.2 Stimulation via Parasympathetic and Sympathetic Nervous Systems

The parotid glands contain only serous cells that produce enzymes and other proteins. The sublingual and submaxillary glands contain both serous and mucous (mucus-producing) cells. In general, the salivary glands produce 1.5 L of saliva per day. Sight, smell, thoughts of food, and food placed in the mouth serve as stimuli for salivation. Both parasympathetic and sympathetic stimulations increase the synthesis and secretion of saliva. Salivary secretion plays a very important role in the maintenance of good oral hygiene because it helps to wash out injurious bacteria and food, neutralize acid, and lubricate food boluses. In addition, saliva initiates triglyceride digestion via *lingual lipase* and starch digestion via *alpha amylase*. Keep in mind that lingual lipase has little functional significance compared to *pancreatic lipase*.

Reality check 4-1: An elderly man presents to the Emergency Department with bradycardia (i.e., a slow pulse rate less than 60 beats/min). Upon review of the patient's medical record, the ER physician notes that in prior visits the patient's bradycardia responded well to the administration of IV *atropine*, an anticholinergic medication. Several minutes after receiving the atropine, the patient complains of a dry mouth. Why?

There are two major stages in the production of saliva. First, acini secrete initial saliva which consists of ptyalin and/or mucin, water, along with ions in a solution that is very similar in composition to extracellular fluid. The ionic composition of the initial saliva is modified as it flows through the salivary ducts (Fig. 4.1b).

The ductal epithelial cells modify the initial saliva through two major active transport processes:

1. Sodium ions (Na^+) are actively reabsorbed and potassium ions (K^+) are actively secreted. Reabsorption of Na^+ exceeds the secretion of K^+ leading to an increased electronegativity of the salivary ducts. Hence, Cl^- ions are reabsorbed passively.
2. Bicarbonate ions (HCO_3^-) are secreted by the ductal epithelial cells.

4.2.3 Contact Theory and Ionic Composition

Basically, there is a net absorption of Na^+ and Cl^- as well as secretion of K^+ and HCO_3^-. The impermeability of the salivary gland ductal cells to water together with the net absorption of solute (NaCl) leads to the production of *hypotonic* final saliva. Salivary composition varies with salivary flow rate. At high flow rates, the salivary ducts have insufficient time to reabsorb NaCl or secrete K^+. In this circumstance the saliva resembles the initial saliva produced by the acinar cells. On the other hand, at the lowest flow rates, the salivary ducts have ample time to reabsorb NaCl and the saliva produced will have a lower concentration of NaCl and a higher concentration of K^+. This contact theory does not hold for HCO_3^- because its secretion is selectively stimulated in parallel with stimulation of saliva production (Fig. 4.2).

4.2.4 Recall Points

Salivary Gland Secretion
- Salivary glands: parotid (serous), sublingual, and submaxillary (serous and mucous).
- Salivary gland secretion is hypotonic.
- Parasympathetic and sympathetic stimulations increase saliva secretion.
- Net absorption of Na^+ and Cl^- against net secretion of K^+ and HCO_3^-.
- Salivary ducts are impermeable to water.
- Contact theory determines ionic composition except for HCO_3^-.
- Saliva and HCO_3^- secretions are stimulated concurrently.

4.3 Gastric Secretions

Composition of Gastric Juice: Gastric juice includes four major constituents: hydrochloric acid (HCl), intrinsic factor, pepsinogen, and mucus. Mucus secreting cells line the entire surface of the stomach. These cells form a protective gel on the

Fig. 4.2 The effect of salivary flow rate on the ionic concentration of saliva. Concentrations of the principal ions, Na^+, HCO_3^-, Cl^-, and K^+, are shown relative to the saliva flow rate. The normal adult plasma concentrations for these ions are $[Na^+]$: 135–145 mM; $[HCO_3^-]$: 22–29 mM; $[Cl^-]$: 95–108 mM; and $[K^+]$: 3.5–5 mM

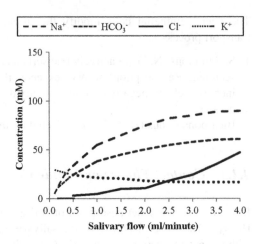

gastric mucosa to protect against the corrosive action of HCl and to lubricate foodstuffs. The two types of tubular glands found in the stomach are the oxyntic and pyloric glands (mucus forming). The *oxyntic glands* contain *parietal* (oxyntic) cells that secrete HCl and *intrinsic factor*, chief (peptic) cells that secrete *pepsinogen*, and *mucus* secreting cells (Fig. 4.3). Acid secreted by the parietal cells activates pepsinogen to pepsin (a protease) via autocatalysis in the gastric lumen and initiates the digestion of proteins by causing them to denature. In addition, the parietal cells secrete intrinsic factor, which forms a complex with vitamin B12 that is later absorbed in the ileum. Intrinsic factor is the only essential component of the gastric juice. The chief cells, which are located deeper in the oxyntic gland, secrete only pepsinogen. The pyloric glands possess a configuration similar to the oxyntic glands. However the pyloric glands have deeper pits and primarily secrete mucus as well as the hormone gastrin. Additionally, pyloric glands secrete a small amount of pepsinogen.

4.3.1   Regulation of Gastric Acid Secretion

The gastric secretion of HCl serves important functions such as activating pepsinogen to *pepsin* and killing luminal pathogens. The mechanism of HCl production occurs via a series of cellular processes (Fig. 4.4). In the intracellular fluid of the parietal cell, the combination of CO_2 and H_2O is catalyzed by carbonic anhydrase to produce H_2CO_3, which dissociates into H^+ and HCO_3^-. The H^+–K^+ ATPase pump located in the apical (luminal) side of the parietal cell secretes H^+ into the gastric lumen. Chloride ion diffuses through Cl^- channels in the apical membrane and follows H^+ into the lumen. In addition, HCO_3^- absorbed into the bloodstream ("the alkaline tide") exchanges for Cl^- via a Cl^-–HCO_3^- exchanger.

Reality check 4-2: After a meal, the gastric venous blood increases in pH. Why?

Fig. 4.3 Gastric oxyntic
gland. Parietal cells secrete
HCl and intrinsic factor,
chief cells secrete
pepsinogen, and mucous
cells secrete mucus

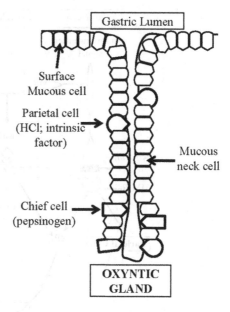

Fig. 4.4 Mechanism of
HCl secretion by the
parietal (oxyntic) cells. *ATP*
Na–K ATPase pump, *CA*
carbonic anhydrase

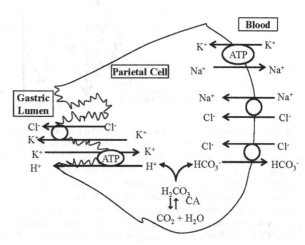

Acetylcholine (ACh), gastrin, and histamine stimulate parietal cells to secrete
H$^+$ (Fig. 4.5). The vagus nerve releases the neurotransmitter ACh, which stimulates
the M$_3$ *muscarinic receptor* on the parietal cell. ACh acts via an IP$_3$/Ca^{2+} second
messenger system to stimulate H$^+$ secretion.

The vagus nerve also innervates G cells via the neurotransmitter gastrin-
releasing peptide (GRP), which stimulates the secretion of gastrin and the subsequent secretion of H$^+$ by an endocrine process (Fig. 4.5). Hence, vagal stimulation
of H$^+$ secretion occurs via both direct and indirect mechanisms. Anticholinergic or
antimuscarinic agents (e.g., atropine) block the direct pathway of vagal stimulation

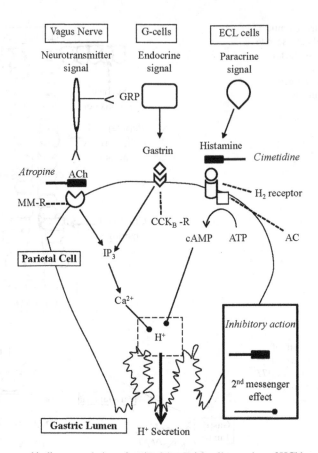

Fig. 4.5 Direct and indirect regulation of parietal (oxyntic) cell secretion of HCl by acetylcholine, gastrin, and histamine, and the inhibitory roles of atropine and cimetidine. Note the direct and indirect effect of vagus nerve stimulation by acetylcholine (ACh) and gastrin-releasing peptide (GRP), respectively, the latter activating gastrin release from G-cells. Acetylcholine, a neurotransmitter, acts via inositol triphosphate (IP_3) and then Ca^{2+} as second messengers to cause H^+ secretion to the gastric lumen after binding to the M_3 muscarinic receptor (MM-R). This action can be blocked by atropine. Gastrin, an endocrine agent, also acts via IP_3–Ca^{2+} after binding to the cholecystokinin$_B$-receptor (CCK_B-R). Histamine, a paracrine agent released by enterochromaffin-like (ECL) cells, binds to a H_2 receptor to activate formation of cyclic AMP (cAMP) from ATP catalyzed by adenylyl cyclase (AC). Histamine action is blocked by cimetidine

of H^+ secretion because ACh is the neurotransmitter. However, atropine does not block the indirect pathway of vagal stimulation of H^+ secretion because GRP is the neurotransmitter. Gastrin is released in response to consuming a meal because of gastric distention, the presence of small peptides, and vagal stimulation. Gastrin binds to the CCK_B (cholecystokinin) receptor of the parietal cell resulting in stimulation of H^+ secretion via the IP_3/Ca^{2+} system. Gastric mucosal enterochromaffin-like (ECL) cells release *histamine*, a paracrine agent, which diffuses a short distance to the parietal cells. Histamine binding to the H_2 receptor promotes H^+ secretion via the second messenger cAMP. Drugs such as *cimetidine* inhibit the secretion of H^+ due to histamine because they are H_2 receptor blocking agents.

H^+ secretion is also regulated by the interaction of ACh, gastrin, and histamine by a process called potentiation. When two stimuli combine to produce a response greater than the sum of their individual responses, then potentiation is said to have occurred. Possible explanations for potentiation during the stimulation of the parietal cell and the production of H^+ include:

1. The stimulation of different receptors which result in the secretion of H^+.
2. Both ACh and gastrin cause ECL cells to release histamine which stimulates H^+ secretion.

Reality check 4-3: Explain the effectiveness of H_2 receptor blocking agents in treating peptic ulcers.

The stimulation of HCl secretion is related to the presence of chyme in the stomach and the need to activate pepsinogen to pepsin. Food serves as a buffer for stomach acid. When food leaves the stomach, the amount of buffer present is reduced. A decrease of the gastric pH to below 3 with the reduction of buffer leads to an inhibition of H^+ secretion. Both direct and indirect pathways for the inhibition of H^+ occur via the action of somatostatin, which is a major inhibitory mechanism for H^+ secretion by parietal cells. Somatostatin binding to receptors on the parietal cell during the direct pathway reduces the amount of cAMP produced by adenylyl cyclase and thus impedes histamine's stimulation of H^+ secretion. Somatostatin impedes the release of gastrin and histamine and hence decreases H^+ secretion by an indirect pathway. Similarly, prostaglandins activate a G_i protein, which inhibits adenylyl cyclase leading to antagonism of histamine's stimulation of H^+ secretion. Nonsteroidal anti-inflammatory drugs (NSAIDs) cause peptic ulcers and retard the healing of ulcers due to their antiprostaglandin effects. Essentially, NSAIDs reduce the action of an inhibitor of gastric acid secretion (prostaglandins) resulting in increased acid production and subsequent mucosal ulceration.

4.3.2   Ulcers

Peptic ulcers are excoriated areas of the GI mucosa which result from either an imbalance between too much H^+ and pepsin secretion and/or the diminution in the amount of HCO_3^- and mucus which normally form a protective mucous barrier. Two-thirds of all ulcers are due to the *H. pylori* bacterium and essentially one-third are related to the use of NSAIDs. Gastric ulcers are basically produced as a result of a defect in the mucosal barrier that causes the digestion of involved mucosa by H^+ and pepsin. The gram negative bacterium, *H. pylori*, is one of the major causes of gastric ulcers because it attaches to the gastric epithelium and releases cytotoxins that damage the epithelial cells and protective mucus layer. *H. pylori* contains an enzyme called urease, which generates NH_3 from urea that in turn causes the local mucous layer to become alkaline. Some neutralization of acid by the ammonia creates a more favorable environment for *H. pylori* compared to the less accommodating acidic gastric pH. *H. pylori* paradoxically induces inflammation and epithelial cell damage in the host without conferring immunity to infection. *H. pylori* infection recruits and activates monocytes and neutrophils by causing an increase in IL-1, IL-6, IL-8, and tumor necrosis factor-alpha (TNF-alpha). The release of the neutrophil mediators disrupts epithelial cells leading to ulcer formation. In addition, *H. pylori* may induce B-cell-mediated autoimmune responses and induce gastritis (inflammation of the stomach mucosal lining).

Reality check 4-4: Patients with gastric ulcers in general have net H^+ secretory rates lower than normal. Why? Gastric ulcer patients also have an increased rate of gastrin. Why?

An oversupply of H^+ in patients with a duodenal ulcer injures the mucosa. In these patients, the gastrin concentration in response to a meal will frequently be increased, although their baseline concentration may be normal. *H. pylori* represents an important etiologic agent in the majority of duodenal ulcers. *H. pylori* inhibits the secretion of somatostatin, an inhibitor of H^+ secretion. Hence, gastric secretion of H^+ is stimulated. In addition, production of both basal and stimulated HCO_3^- in the proximal duodenum markedly diminishes in patients with active duodenal ulcers. In contrast, distal duodenal HCO_3^- production remains normal. The exact mechanism of this defect is still under investigation.

Reality check 4-5: Briefly describe the mechanism of action of the following drugs that block gastric H^+ secretion:

(a) Atropine (antimuscarinic agent)
(b) Cimetidine (H_2 receptor blocking agent)
(c) *Omeprazole* (H^+, K^+-ATPase inhibitor)

4.3.3   Recall Points

Gastric Secretions
- Major components of gastric juice: HCl, intrinsic factor, pepsinogen, and mucus.
- Acetylcholine and gastrin stimulate the parietal cell via IP_3/Ca^{2+}.
- Histamine stimulates the parietal cell via cAMP.
- Stimulation of HCl is related to the presence of chyme in the stomach.
- H^+ secretion is also regulated by the interaction of ACh, gastrin, and histamine by a process called potentiation.
- Two-thirds of all peptic ulcers are caused by *H. pylori* and one-third of all ulcers are due to NSAIDs.
- Gastric ulcers are basically produced due to a defect in the mucosal barrier leading to digestion of the involved mucosa by H^+ and pepsin.
- Duodenal ulcer patient's mucosa is injured by an oversupply of H^+.

4.4   Pancreatic Secretions

4.4.1   Acinar Versus Ductal Cell Contributions

The pancreas, a compound gland, consists of an endocrine and an exocrine portion. The exocrine portion of the pancreas secretes about 1 L of isotonic fluid per 24 h. The anatomy of the exocrine pancreas (Fig. 4.6) is similar to that of the salivary gland (cf. Fig. 4.1a) because it consists of an acinus, which is the blind end of a branching ductular system. The acinar cells secrete pancreatic digestive enzymes and the centroacinar and ductal cells secrete HCO_3^- (Fig. 4.6). In contrast to salivary gland secretion, the parasympathetic nervous system stimulates pancreatic secretion, whereas the sympathetic nervous system decreases pancreatic secretion largely by changing blood flow away from the pancreas. The pancreas secretes enzymes responsible for the digestion of carbohydrates, proteins, and lipids. Centroacinar and *ductal cells* secrete water and HCO_3^-, the other key components of pancreatic secretion. Pancreatic amylase, which aids digestion of carbohydrates, pancreatic lipase, which facilitates digestion of lipids, cholesterol esterase, which hydrolyzes cholesterol esters, and phospholipase, which removes fatty acids from phospholipids, are secreted in inactive forms.

4.4.2   Pancreatic Protease Activation

Pancreatic proteases, which are responsible for the digestion of proteins, are secreted into the intestinal lumen as inactive precursors. These inactive proteolytic enzyme precursors include *trypsinogen*, chymotrypsinogen, and procarboxy-peptidase, which become activated in the gut lumen. For example, trypsinogen is activated by the duodenal brush border enzyme enteropeptidase to become trypsin. *Trypsin* will then activate chymotrypsinogen to chymotrypsin, procarboxy-peptidase to carboxypeptidase, proelastase to elastase, and trypsinogen to trypsin. Acute pancreatitis occurs when there is autodigestion of pancreatic cells because of the premature activation of trypsinogen within the pancreas and thus initiation of the cascade activating the other proteases. Several mechanisms normally prevent the premature activation of trypsinogen including synthesis of pancreatic inhibitors, *zymogen* separation from lysosomes, and the ability of trypsin, when it contacts other trypsin molecules, to irreversibly inactivate them.

4.4.3   Regulation of Pancreatic Secretions

Entry of small peptides, amino acids, and fatty acids into the duodenum triggers the release of CCK by I cells. CCK stimulates secretion of digestive enzymes from the

Fig. 4.6 Structure of the exocrine pancreas. The acini contain acinar cells, which secrete enzymes responsible for digestion of starch, lipids, and protein. The acini also contain centroacinar cells that along with the ductal cells secrete bicarbonate and water. The parasympathetic nervous system (PNS) stimulates secretion. The sympathetic nervous system (SNS) counterbalances this PNS effect by diverting blood flow away from the pancreas

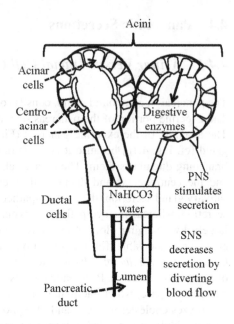

pancreas as well as bile acids from the gall bladder. Entry of H^+ into the duodenum triggers the release of secretin by the S cells resulting in the ductal cells secreting HCO_3^- ions to neutralize the H^+ present in the lumen. Acetylcholine further aids in these events by stimulating pancreatic enzyme secretion and potentiating the action of secretin. Its release via vagovagal reflexes occurs in response to H^+, fatty acids, peptides, and small amino acids in the lumen of the duodenum.

The HCO_3^- and Cl^- ion concentrations of pancreatic juice vary with the flow rate in an inverse manner owing to the action of the Cl^-/HCO_3^- exchanger in the apical border of the ductal cells. At high flow rates the pancreatic juice contains the highest HCO_3^- ion concentration relative to Cl^- ion concentration. The opposite is true for low flow rates.

Reality check 4-6: Cystic fibrosis (CF) is caused by a defect in Cl^- transport and water flux across the apical surface of epithelial cells. Abnormally thick mucus is produced by most of the exocrine glands and ducts. Hence, cystic fibrosis affects not only the pancreas but also the intestinal mucosa, the sweat glands, and the respiratory epithelium (the most serious effect). CF patients experience chronic lung disease and pancreatic insufficiency. Why would these patients develop diarrhea and malabsorption?

4.4.4   Recall Points

Pancreatic Secretion
• Acinar cells secrete the enzymatic portion of pancreatic secretion.
• Centroacinar and ductal cells secrete HCO_3^-.

- Pancreatic proteases are secreted as inactive precursors.
- Pancreatic secretion is isotonic.
- Parasympathetic nervous system stimulates pancreatic secretion.
- Sympathetic nervous system decreases pancreatic secretion.
- Concentrations of HCO_3^- and Cl^- ion concentrations vary relative to each other in an inverse manner depending on the flow rate and the action of the Cl^-–HCO_3^- exchanger.

4.5 Biliary Secretions

Synthesis and Secretion of Bile Acids and Salts: Bile, produced by the hepatocytes, is composed of bile salts, phospholipids, cholesterol, bile pigments, water, and ions. The liver continuously synthesizes bile from cholesterol and the bile drains into the bile ducts for storage in the gallbladder. Primary bile acids (cholic acid and chenodeoxycholic acid) are produced in the liver from cholesterol. Secondary bile acids (deoxycholic and lithocholic) are produced when bacteria metabolize primary bile acids in the gut lumen. Bile salts are formed when bile acids are conjugated with either glycine or taurine. Bile salts have a lower (more acidic) pK than bile acids; 1–4 compared to 7. According to the Henderson–Hasselbalch equation where $pH = pK + log[A^-/HA]$, a strong acid (i.e., one with a lower pK) ionizes sooner than a weaker acid (i.e., one with a higher pK) as the local pH becomes more alkaline. Hence stronger acids ionize more readily. Therefore in the duodenal lumen where the pH is 3–5, bile salts will be in their ionized form (A^-) and will be more water soluble than will their bile acid counterparts.

The liver not only secretes the bile it produces (Fig. 4.7) but also the bile that recirculates via *enterohepatic circulation* (Fig. 4.8). About 75 % of intestinal bile salts are reabsorbed in the ileum and returned to the liver for secretion. The gallbladder concentrates bile and stores it for release with meals. During the interdigestive period, the sphincter of Oddi is contracted and the gallbladder is relaxed which allows it to fill. The gallbladder concentrates bile by absorbing water and ions. Bile is ejected from the gallbladder within 30 min of ingesting a meal. In addition to fatty acids and protein digestion products causing CCK release and thus stimulating gallbladder contraction and the release of bile to facilitate lipid absorption, this concurrently promotes pancreatic acinar cell release of proteolytic enzymes to deal with the protein component of the diet (Fig. 4.7).

Role of Micelles in Lipid Absorption: How do bile salts aid in the absorption of lipids? Bile salts are amphipathic because they have both hydrophilic (water soluble) and hydrophobic (lipid soluble) sections. Above a critical concentration, bile salts form micelles. The bile salts emulsify various products of lipid digestion that aggregate in the center of the mixed micelle. These products include 2-monoacylglycerol, formed by removal of two fatty acids by lipolysis of triglyceride catalyzed by pancreatic lipase, cholesterol derived from cholesterol ester via cholesterol esterase, and lysolecithin that originates from phospholipid via

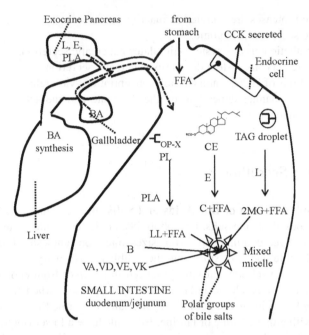

Fig. 4.7 Digestion of lipids in the small intestine. The lipids digested include triglyceride (TAG) in droplets converted into 2-monoacylglycerol (MG) and 2 free fatty acids (FFA) by pancreatic lipase (L), cholesterol ester (CE) converted into cholesterol (C) and FFA by cholesterol esterase (E), and phospholipids (PL) converted into lysolecithin (LL) and FFA by phospholipase A2 (PLA). These products together with fat soluble vitamins A, D, E, and K (VA, VD, VE, VK) are emulsified by bile salts (B), which are derived from bile acids (BA) produced by the liver, to generate mixed micelles. Cholecystokinin (CCK), which is released from intestinal endocrine cells by FFA derived from the stomach, stimulates the pancreas to secrete its digestive enzymes and the gallbladder (GB) to contract to release its bile acid stores

phospholipase A_2, with the latter two reactions releasing a single fatty acid. The fat soluble vitamins aggregate in the center of the mixed micelle as well (Fig. 4.7).

Polar groups of the bile salts line the surface of the micelle making the micelle water soluble so that it can interact with the brush border of intestinal cells. Hence, the lipid products of digestion can dissolve in the aqueous environment. This process is necessary because of the unstirred water layer that sits on top of the microvilli. If this aqueous barrier was not present then bile salt micelles with a lipid core would not be required at this stage in the process. The micelles transport the lipid products of digestion to the apical membrane of the intestinal epithelial cells where the digested products are released and diffuse into the cells (Fig. 4.8).

Processing of Absorbed Lipids: Once inside the intestinal cells, the lipid digestion products (i.e., 2-monoacylglycerol, cholesterol, and lysolecithin) are reesterified with free fatty acids to form triacylglycerol (containing long-chain fatty acids), cholesterol ester, and phospholipids, respectively, which combine with apoproteins to form lipid-transporting particles called *chylomicrons*

Fig. 4.8 Lipid absorption, reesterification, and incorporation into chylomicrons in the small intestine. Mixed micelles release their contents that enter intestinal epithelial cells. Bile salts are recirculated from the ileum to the liver via the enterohepatic circulation. *C* cholesterol, *CE* cholesterol ester, *FFA* free fatty acid, *MG* 2-monoacylglycerol, *LL* lysolecithin, *PL* phospholipid, *TG* triglyceride, *VA* vitamin A, *VD* vitamin D, *VE* vitamin E, *VK* vitamin K

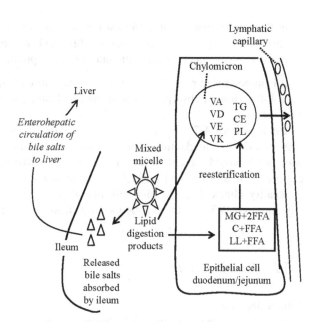

(Fig. 4.8). The chylomicrons move to the basolateral portion of the intestinal epithelial cell and undergo exocytosis. Because of their large size, the chylomicrons enter the lymphatic capillaries rather than the vascular capillaries. After entering the lymphatic circulation, the chylomicrons pass to the thoracic duct which empties into the blood.

Problems with lipid absorption may occur due to the following causes:

1. Insufficiency of the exocrine pancreas leads to decreased production of pancreatic enzymes (i.e., lipase, phospholipase A_2, and cholesterol ester hydrolase). When the patient has a deficiency of pancreatic lipase, triglycerides cannot be digested into monoglycerides and free fatty acids. The unabsorbed triglycerides cause steatorrhea, which is increased excretion of fat in the stools.
2. An interruption of the enterohepatic circulation, whether due to removal/effacement of the terminal ileum or decrease in bile salts, interferes with the formation of bile salts and the subsequent absorption of the breakdown products of lipid digestion.
3. Decreased intestinal absorptive area either due to surgical resection or due to destruction of intestinal epithelial cells from any cause significantly reduces the available surface for intestinal absorption of lipids.
4. Hyperacidity of duodenal contents decreases activity of pancreatic enzymes and reduces absorption of lipids.
5. Overgrowth of bacteria results in the deconjugation of bile salts and the malabsorption of lipids. Deconjugation of bile salts (i.e., removal of glycine and taurine) reverts them to bile acids. The pK of bile acids being higher than that of the intestinal lumen prevents the bile acids from ionizing so that they remain

in their more lipid soluble (less water soluble) form in which they are easily absorbed. The premature absorption of bile acids before they reach the terminal ileum reduces micelle formation and lipid absorption.

It is important to note that regardless of the cause of impaired lipid absorption, fat soluble vitamin absorption also decreases leading to a potential deficiency of each vitamin.

Reality check 4-7: *Crohn's disease* is an inflammatory bowel disorder in which patients exhibit a thickening of their mucosa and all other layers of the intestinal wall. Why would patients with Crohn's disease involving their terminal ileum experience steatorrhea and suffer from malabsorption?

Reality check 4-8: Patients with *abetalipoproteinemia* are not able to form chylomicrons. Why do these patients suffer from steatorrhea?

4.5.1 Recall Points

Biliary Secretion
- Primary bile acids (cholic and chenodeoxycholic acid), secondary bile acids (deoxycholic and lithocholic acid).
- Bile salts form by conjugation of bile acids with glycine or taurine.
- Bile salts have a pK 1–4, bile acids have a pK 7, duodenal lumen pK 3–5.
- Bile salts will be in an ionized form (A^-) in the duodenal lumen and will be more water soluble than bile acids.
- Problems with lipid absorption occur due to pancreatic exocrine insufficiency, an interruption of the enterohepatic circulation, decreased intestinal absorptive area, hyperacidity of the duodenal contents, and bacterial overgrowth.

4.6 Intestinal Absorption and Secretion

4.6.1 Absorption

The small and large intestines absorb approximately 9 L of fluid every day. Of this amount, 2 L is derived from dietary sources, while the remainder is from salivary, pancreaticobiliary, gastric, and intestinal secretions. The epithelial cells lining the intestinal villi are very efficient and absorb a large quantity of water, Na^+, Cl^-, HCO_3^-, and K^+. In general, the small and large intestinal villi absorb all but 100–200 mL that eventually is excreted in the stool. The majority of absorption occurs in the small intestine. In contrast, the epithelial cells lining the crypts secrete fluid and electrolytes.

Tight Junctions and Intestinal Permeability: Water and electrolytes travel across intestinal epithelial cells via cellular routes or in between cells via paracellular routes (see Fig. 2.2). Intestinal epithelial cells attach to each other at the luminal membrane. The permeability of the tight junctions of epithelial cells dictates whether electrolytes and water move via cellular or paracellular routes. The *tight junctions* of the small intestine tend to be leaky or permeable and those of the large intestine tend to be tight or impermeable.

Absorption of Na^+ in the small intestine (i.e., jejunum and ileum) occurs primarily by cotransport mechanisms involving glucose or amino acids or by a Na^+/H^+ exchange mechanism (Fig. 4.9a, b). The glucose and amino acids then pass through the basolateral membrane into the blood. The H^+ is derived from the splitting of H_2CO_3 by carbonic anhydrase (see Fig. 4.4) with the HCO_3^- either transported to the blood out of the jejunal epithelial cell (Fig. 4.9a) or exchanged for absorbed Cl^- in the ileal epithelial cell (Fig. 4.9b). The absorption of Cl^- by the jejunum also coincides with Na^+ but occurs by paracellular passive diffusion (Fig. 4.9a). The Na^+–K^+ ATPase pump located in the basolateral membrane pumps Na^+ out of the cell against its electrochemical gradient in exchange for K^+.

Sodium and Potassium: In the colon, the most important mechanism for the absorption of Na^+ occurs via passive diffusion through Na^+ channels whose numbers can be increased by the action of aldosterone (Fig. 4.10). The net absorption of dietary or secretion-derived K^+ occurs by passive diffusion via a paracellular route. Additionally, the colonic apical and basolateral membranes both are permeable to K^+ (not so in the small intestine). Because the Na^+–K^+ pump maintains a high intracellular concentration of K^+, some K^+ passively leaks across the epithelial cell apical membranes. Secretion of K^+ is increased by factors that elevate intracellular K^+ (e.g., aldosterone-stimulated Na^+ absorption) (Fig. 4.10). In addition, the colonic secretion of K^+ increases with the flow rate of stool. This flow rate-dependent mechanism is similar to what is found in the distal renal tubule. When patients suffer from the rapid passage of diarrheal stools, they experience intravascular volume reduction, which stimulates the secretion of aldosterone. Hence, more K^+ is lost via increased secretion in the stool and the patient may develop hypokalemia. Absorption of chloride in exchange for HCO_3^- occurs in a similar fashion to what takes place in the ileum (see Fig. 4.9b).

Water: Water absorption occurs secondary to solute absorption. In the small intestine and gallbladder, water absorption happens in an isosmotic fashion. The large intestine is less permeable to the movement of water back into the lumen. In fact the "tight epithelium" of the colonic mucosa allows a large transmucosal Na^+ gradient to be established with the concurrent absorption of large quantities of water. In the small intestine, a much smaller transmucosal gradient exists for Na^+ because, if its luminal concentration falls by ~15 mM, the Na^+ is then drawn back into the lumen via the paracellular spaces that exist in this "leaky epithelium." At the same time, water moves back in this direction as a result. Paradoxically although most water absorption occurs in the small intestine, the colon actually carries out this function much more effectively.

Fat Soluble Vitamins: Absorption of the fat soluble vitamins (i.e., A, D, E, and K) occurs in a fashion similar to other dietary lipids via the action of micelles. In contrast, absorption of water soluble vitamins utilizes a Na^+-dependent cotransport

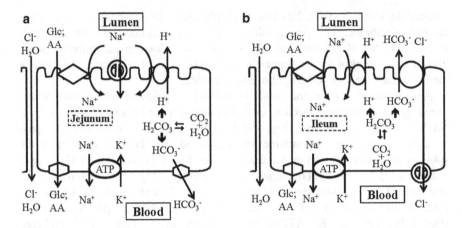

Fig. 4.9 Electrolyte transport in the small intestine. Glucose (Glc) and amino acids (AA) are absorbed via a sodium-dependent process. The sodium electrochemical gradient is maintained by the Na–K ATPase pump (ATP). Sodium also exchanges across the luminal membrane with protons that are produced by the action of carbonic anhydrase that catalyzes the conversion of CO_2 and H_2O to H^+ and HCO_3^- (bicarbonate). (**a**) Jejunum, bicarbonate from carbonic anhydrase, diffuses into the blood. (**b**) Ileum, bicarbonate from carbonic anhydrase, exchanges with chloride, from the intestinal lumen, which in turn diffuses into the blood

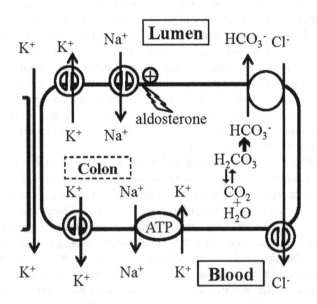

Fig. 4.10 Electrolyte transport in the colon. Sodium influx is stimulated by aldosterone, a mineralocorticoid. As in the ileum, bicarbonate from carbonic anhydrase exchanges with chloride, which then diffuses into the blood. *ATP* Na–K ATPase pump

Fig. 4.11 Calcium
absorption in the intestine.
1,25D₃ active vitamin D,
Ca-ATP Ca-ATPase pump,
CaBP calcium binding
protein, *DBP* vitamin D
binding protein

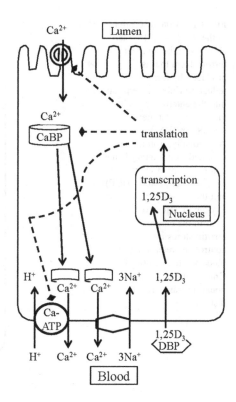

process. Vitamin B12, a water soluble vitamin, is an exception to the rule because it requires binding with intrinsic factor with this complex being absorbed in the terminal ileum.

Calcium: Absorption of Ca^{2+} occurs in the proximal small intestine via vitamin D-dependent calcium binding protein mechanism (Fig. 4.11). Transport of Ca^{2+} increases when active vitamin D_3 ($1,25\text{-}(OH)_2\text{-}D_3$) interacts with enterocyte nuclear receptors causing the synthesis of calcium binding protein (CaBP). CaBP facilitates the entry of Ca^{2+} into the intestinal cell along with an increased number of epithelial Ca^{2+} channels. Subsequently, Ca^{2+} leaves the cell at the basolateral membrane against an electrochemical gradient via two mechanisms: (1) The Ca^{2+}-ATPase, which is the more important mechanism and (2) a Na^+–Ca^{2+} exchange mechanism, which functions when the Ca^{2+}-ATPase becomes saturated. Cytosolic CaBP is believed to also stimulate Ca^+-ATPase. The Golgi, endoplasmic reticulum, and perhaps mitochondrial binding proteins play a key role in preventing the intracellular rise of Ca^{2+} during absorption. A deficiency of vitamin D causes decreased Ca^{2+} absorption that results in rickets in children and osteomalacia in adults.

Iron: Iron plays an important role as a component of many enzymes, as well as in the oxygen binding of hemoglobin. Iron absorption occurs as either its free divalent ferrous (Fe^{2+}) form taken up via the divalent metal transporter or heme iron (i.e., bound to either myoglobin or hemoglobin) (Fig. 4.12). Heme iron taken

Fig. 4.12 Iron absorption in the duodenum. Iron is absorbed in its divalent ferrous form that is produced by ferric reductase (FR). Absorption into the enterocyte occurs via the divalent metal transporter (DMT). Additionally, iron may be obtained from dietary heme that is absorbed via the heme carrier protein (HCP) and then degraded by heme oxygenase (HO) to release iron. In the enterocyte, ferritin stores iron and controls its release into the blood via ferroportin (FP). Once in the blood iron is bound to transferrin for distribution

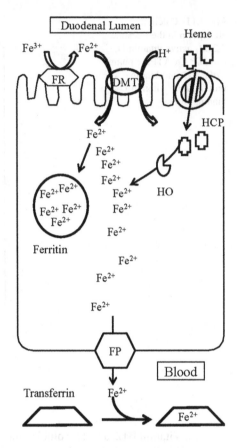

up by the intestinal cells via the heme carrier protein is released as free iron in the cell by an enzymatic process catalyzed by heme oxygenase. Once inside the enterocyte, iron follows one of two major pathways. Which path is taken depends on a complex balance within the cell based on amounts of dietary and systemic iron. When iron is abundant, it is stored in the enterocyte by binding to ferritin. Death of the enterocyte leads to loss of this iron.

In contrast, under circumstances when iron is limiting, it is exported out of the enterocyte via a transporter, ferroportin that is located in the basolateral membrane. Once in the blood, iron binds to a carrier protein, transferrin, for distribution throughout the body.

4.6.2   Diarrhea

The intestinal crypt cells secrete fluid and electrolytes, whereas the cells lining the villi are responsible for absorption of fluids and electrolytes. The basolateral membrane contains both a Na^+–K^+ ATPase and a Na^+–K^+–$2Cl^-$ cotransporter

(Fig. 4.13a). The three ion cotransporter brings Cl^- into the intestinal cell, but Cl^- subsequently leaves the cell by diffusion through apical membrane CFTR-Cl^- channels. Sodium ions passively follow secretion of Cl^- ions via a paracellular route. Water secretion into the lumen follows NaCl secretion. Most of the time, the apical membrane Cl^- channels are closed, but they can be opened in response to the binding of neurotransmitters (ACh and VIP) or hormones to the basolateral membrane receptors thus activating adenylyl cyclase and generating cAMP. The apical membrane Cl^- channels open in response to cAMP, resulting in Cl^- secretion into the lumen, followed by Na^+ and water. Generally, the water and electrolytes secreted by the crypt cells are absorbed by the intestinal villi cells.

Consider the special case of *Vibrio cholerae* or cholera toxin-induced diarrhea, which is due to the excessive stimulation of Cl^- secretion. The cholera toxin permanently activates adenylyl cyclase causing the production and an increase in cAMP intracellular concentration (Fig. 4.13b). cAMP activates protein kinase A, which in turn phosphorylates the CFTR chloride channel that opens. As long as this phosphorylation remains unabated, the channel remains open to allow Cl^- flow into the intestinal lumen. Flow of the chloride anion into the lumen attracts the sodium cation to enter the lumen by a paracellular route. Water also enters because of the high electrolyte concentration in the lumen. The Na^+ and water following Cl^- into the lumen results in a secretory diarrhea. Hence adenylyl cyclase activity is sustained which results in large amounts of intestinal fluid secretion that overwhelms the absorptive capacity of the villi. Patients suffering from cholera toxin-induced diarrhea may become severely volume contracted and at risk of death. Oral rehydration therapy effectively treats cholera because of the use of substrate-coupled cotransport of Na^+ and glucose by enterocytes to absorb water and thus oppose the water loss occurring via crypt cell Cl^- secretion.

Case in Point 4-1

Chief Complaint: Heartburn, epigastric abdominal pain, and diarrhea.

History: A 39-year-old man presents with epigastric abdominal pain, heartburn, and diarrhea. He has failed a 2 week trial of a proton pump inhibitor. GI review of symptoms is also significant for decreased appetite, 12 lb weight loss in the last month, and black stools.

Physical Exam: A middle-aged man appearing chronically ill and in moderate distress. Vital signs are temperature 99.6 °F, blood pressure 100/60 mmHg, pulse 110/min, and respirations 18/min. Physical examination of the skin reveals decreased turgor. Abdominal exam reveals tenderness to palpation in the midepigastrium, hyperactive bowel sounds, and black stools on digital exam. The rest of the exam is unremarkable.

Labs:

Hematocrit 34 % (normal: 41–50 %), low mean corpuscular volume.

Leukocytes (white blood cells) $12 \times 10^3/\mu L$ (normal: 3.8–10.8×10^3) without a left shift.

(continued)

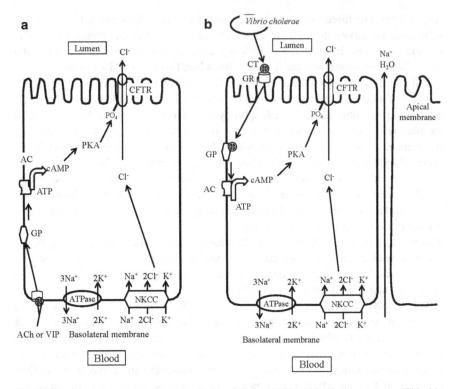

Fig. 4.13 Chloride transport across the apical membrane. (**a**) Normal chloride transport. Chloride channels are opened by the action of neurotransmitters acetylcholine (ACh) or vasoactive intestinal peptide (VIP) acting via G-protein (GP) to activate adenylyl cyclase (AC). AC produces cAMP that activates protein kinase A (PKA), which phosphorylates and thus opens the CFTR (cystic fibrosis transmembrane conductance regulator) chloride channel. Intracellular sodium and potassium are regulated by the Na–K ATPase (ATPase) and the sodium–potassium–chloride cotransporter (NKCC). The latter also brings chloride into the cell that can be secreted via the CFTR. (**b**) Mechanism of cholera toxin-induced diarrhea due to excessive chloride transport. A toxin (CT) produced by *V. cholera* binds to a ganglioside receptor (GR) on the apical membrane. The toxin is internalized into the enterocyte where it activates the sequence leading to unabated phosphorylation of CFTR

Chemistry panel, liver function tests/amylase, and lipase are normal.

Stool guaiac positive for occult blood. Results of recent esophagogastroduodenoscopy reveal multiple gastric and duodenal ulcers. Serum gastrin level of 5,000 off proton pump inhibitor (normal: <100 pg/mL). Abdominal CT revealed a 2 cm well circumscribed pancreatic head mass compatible with a gastrinoma (gastrin secreting tumor).

Assessment: On the basis of these findings, why does this patient experience abdominal pain, diarrhea, weight loss, and anemia?

Reality check 4-9: Imagine that a 675 lb patient comes to your office concerning a second opinion about GI bypass surgery. The patient's records indicate that the bariatric surgeon plans to perform a bypass from the stomach to the distal terminal ileum, effectively bypassing over 70 % of the small intestine. The patient wants to know what types of long-term problems he may face after the surgery.

4.6.3 Recall Points

Intestinal Absorption and Secretion
- Epithelial cells lining the villi absorb large quantities of water, Na^+, Cl^-, HCO_3^-, and K^+.
- Epithelial cells lining the crypts secrete fluid and electrolytes.
- Tight junctions of the small intestine are leaky (permeable).
- Tight junctions of the large intestine are tight (impermeable).
- Absorption of NaCl in the proximal small intestine occurs by involving Na^+–glucose cotransport, Na^+–amino acid cotransport, or by a Na^+–H^+ exchange.
- Na^+–K^+ ATPase pump in the basolateral membrane pumps Na^+ out against its electrochemical gradient.
- Absorption of Cl^- occurs by Na^+–Cl^- cotransport, passive diffusion, or Cl^-–HCO_3^- exchange.
- The most important mechanism for Na^+ absorption in the colon is passive diffusion through Na^+ channels.
- Dietary K^+ absorption occurs by passive diffusion via a paracellular route.
- Potassium ion is actively secreted in the colon by a process which is stimulated by aldosterone.

Connecting-the-Dots 4-1

A 46-year-old man with chronic pancreatitis and pancreatic insufficiency comes to see you in the office. The patient indicates that he has aggravation of abdominal pain with food ingestion and has experienced a significant decrease in his appetite due to the fear of exacerbating the pain. In addition, he complains of weight loss, diarrhea, and steatorrhea (increased fat excretion in the stools). The patient has imbibed 2 six packs of beer per day for the past 20 years. When you examine his abdomen, you note a tender fullness and palpable mass in the epigastrium, suggesting the presence of a pseudocyst or an inflammatory pancreatic mass in the abdomen. In addition, you note decreased subcutaneous fat, temporal wasting, sunken supraclavicular fossa, and other physical signs of malnutrition. What are the likely physiological causes of his symptoms?

4.7   Summary Points

- The parotid (serous), submaxillary, and sublingual (serous and mucus producing) are the three sets of paired salivary glands.
- An increase in the synthesis and secretion of saliva is caused by both parasympathetic and sympathetic nervous system stimulation.
- Concerning salivary secretion, the contact theory holds that the absorption of Na^+ and Cl^-, as well as the secretion of K^+ in the salivary duct, increases with increased contact time.
- Both parasympathetic and sympathetic stimulations lead to an increase in the synthesis and secretion of saliva.
- Salivary HCO_3^- secretion increases when salivary secretion flow increases and secretion decreases when salivary secretion flow decreases.
- The main components of gastric juice are HCl, pepsinogen, mucus, and intrinsic factor.
- Acid or oxyntic glands secrete HCl, intrinsic factor, mucus, and pepsinogen.
- Pyloric glands primarily secrete mucus in addition to gastrin.
- HCl secretion by the stomach serves to activate pepsinogen to pepsin and to kill luminal pathogens.
- The parietal cells are stimulated to secrete H^+ by acetylcholine, gastrin, and histamine.
- Both ACh and gastrin act via an IP_3/Ca^{2+} second messenger system to stimulate H^+ secretion.
- cAMP is the second messenger involved in the stimulation of H^+ secretion by histamine.
- H^+ secretion is also regulated by the interaction of ACh, gastrin, and histamine by a process called potentiation.
- Gastrin and ACh both cause ECL cells to release histamine and induce H^+ secretion by an indirect mechanism.
- The binding of somatostatin to receptors on the parietal cell decreases adenylyl cyclase levels and decreases histamine stimulation of H^+.
- *H. pylori* causes 2/3 of all peptic ulcers, NSAIDs cause approximately 1/3 of all peptic ulcers.
- A gastric ulcer is a defect in the mucosal barrier which results from the digestion of the involved mucosa by H^+ and pepsin.
- Duodenal ulcer patients' mucosa is injured by an oversupply of H^+.
- Sympathetic nervous system decreases pancreatic exocrine secretion; the parasympathetic nervous system stimulates pancreatic exocrine secretion.
- The secretion of pancreatic proteases occurs initially in the form of inactive precursors.
- Entry of amino acids, small peptides, and fatty acids into the duodenum triggers CCK release by the I cells leading to pancreatic enzyme secretion.

- The entry of H^+ into the duodenum causes secretin to be secreted by the S cells leading to the pancreatic ductal cells secreting HCO_3^- to neutralize the H^+ present in the lumen.
- The Cl^-–HCO_3^- exchanger in the apical border of the pancreatic ductal cells causes the concentrations of HCO_3^- and Cl^- in pancreatic juice to vary inversely with the flow rate.
- The liver produces the primary bile acids (cholic and chenodeoxycholic acid) from cholesterol.
- Bacteria metabolize primary bile acids in the gut lumen to produce secondary bile acids (deoxycholic and lithocholic acid).
- Conjugation of bile acids with either glycine or taurine forms bile salts.
- The respective pK of bile salts and bile acids is 1–4 and 7 compared to a pH of 3–5 in the duodenal lumen.
- Bile salts in the duodenal lumen tend to be in their ionized (A^-) form and hence are more water soluble.
- Lipid absorption may be compromised by insufficiency of the exocrine pancreas, interruption of the enterohepatic circulation, hyperacidity of duodenal contents, decreased intestinal absorptive area, and/or bacterial overgrowth.
- The tight junctions of the colon are less leaky than those of the small intestine.
- NaCl absorption in the proximal portion of the small intestine is mediated via cotransport mechanisms involving Na^+–glucose, Na^+–amino acid, or by Na^+–H^+ exchange.
- The Na^+–K^+ ATPase pump located in the basolateral membrane of the parietal cell is responsible for pumping Na^+ out of the cell against its electrochemical gradient.
- Cl^- absorption accompanies Na^+ absorption and occurs by Na^+–Cl^- cotransport, passive diffusion, or Cl^-–HCO_3^- exchange.
- The most important mechanism for the colonic absorption of Na^+ is passive diffusion through Na^+ channels.
- Dietary K^+ absorption occurs by passive diffusion via a paracellular route.
- Aldosterone stimulates colonic secretion of K^+.
- The rate of colonic K^+ secretion is directly proportional to the flow rate of stool.
- Water soluble vitamin absorption in the intestine is mediated by a Na^+-dependent cotransport.
- Vitamin B12 is a water soluble vitamin which requires binding to intrinsic factor rather than Na^+-dependent cotransport.
- Ca^{2+} absorption in the small intestine is mediated by a vitamin D-dependent calcium binding protein mechanism.
- The duodenum is the primary site of iron absorption.
- Cholera toxin induces diarrhea by activating adenylyl cyclase and subsequently cAMP levels which results in an opening of Cl^- channels in the luminal membrane.

4.8 Review Questions

4-1. A 60-year-old patient is prescribed pilocarpine, a cholinergic agonist, for increased ocular pressure. The patient subsequently experiences a very rapid salivary flow rate. You measure the composition of the patient's saliva. Knowing that salivary composition is governed by the contact theory, which of the following statements is correct regarding the reabsorption of NaCl and secretion of K^+ by the salivary ducts?

A. At high flow rates, the salivary ducts reabsorb less NaCl or secrete less K^+
B. At high flow rates, the salivary ducts reabsorb more NaCl or secrete less K^+
C. At high flow rates, the salivary ducts reabsorb the same amount of NaCl or secrete more K^+
D. At low flow rates, the salivary ducts reabsorb less NaCl or secrete more K^+

4-2. A middle-aged man underwent a total gastrectomy for stomach cancer. Because of the surgical removal of his stomach, which of the following supplement schemes will this patient require?

A. Injection of pepsin
B. Injection of vitamin B12
C. Pepsin by mouth
D. Vitamin B12 by mouth

4-3. During the control arm of an experiment, you perform pancreatic function testing on a normal volunteer. Intravenous administration of which substance is correctly paired with an appropriate response?

A. Administration of cholecystokinin (CCK) decreases pancreatic enzyme secretion
B. Administration of cholecystokinin (CCK) elicits no effect on pancreatic enzyme secretion
C. Administration of secretin decreases pancreatic bicarbonate secretion
D. Administration of secretin increases pancreatic bicarbonate secretion

4-4. You have synthesized a very palatable bile salt from cholic acid called supraglycocholic acid (SGC). You plan to corner the bile salt replacement market with your preparation. The pK of SGC is 2, pK of cholic acid is 7, pK of duodenal lumen is 3–5. When the bile salt SGC is present in the duodenal lumen, which of the following statements is most likely to be true?

A. SGC will be in its ionized form and will be more water soluble
B. SGC will be in its ionized form and will not be more water soluble
C. SGC will be in its nonionized form and will be more water soluble
D. SGC will be in its nonionized form and will not be more water soluble

4-5. Sodium can be absorbed in the colon. Which of the following is the primary mechanism by which absorption of Na^+ occurs?

    A. Cotransport with amino acids
    B. Cotransport with glucose
    C. Exchange with H^+
    D. Passive diffusion

4.9 Answer to Case in Point

Case in Point 4-1: Zollinger–Ellison syndrome (ZES) is a disorder in which a tumor in the pancreas or small intestine produces increased amounts of the hormone gastrin that circulates in the blood. ZES patients develop an ulcer diathesis (i.e., predisposition) due to hypersecretion of acid. The increased amount of acid over-rides the ability of the stomach and duodenum to buffer the acid. Hence, these patients experience pain due to severe ulcer disease, which may lead to decreased appetite, reduced weight, and black stools due to upper gastrointestinal bleeding.

ZES patients may experience diarrhea due to the voluminous amounts of gastric juice secretion that contains acid. The intestinal capacity to absorb the fluid is exceeded resulting in diarrhea. The large acidic fluid load inactivates pancreatic enzymes thereby impeding the digestion of dietary lipids. Additionally, in the more acidic environment in the intestinal lumen of these patients the bile salts, which are weak acids, revert to their nonionized form. In their nonionized form, they become lipid soluble and consequently are absorbed by the proximal small intestine before the formation of micelles and the absorption of lipids can be completed. This decrease of intestinal bile salts results in increased fat in stools (steatorrhea), diarrhea and weight loss.

ZES patients may present with anemia due to intestinal bleeding, malabsorption, and nutritional deficiencies as indicated above.

4.10 Answer to Connecting-the-Dots

Connecting-the-Dots 4-1: Chronic pancreatitis results from severe inflammation of the pancreas and is caused by excessive alcohol consumption in ~70 % of the cases in the USA. The pancreas is a resilient organ because pancreatic insufficiency is generally not seen until 90 % of the organ is damaged. The pancreas secretes enzymes responsible for the digestion of carbohydrates, proteins, and lipids. Other key components of pancreatic secretion include water and HCO_3^-. The patient's abdominal pain is aggravated with food ingestion because food in the stomach, and subsequently in the duodenum, triggers pancreatic secretion. In the face of a swollen pancreas this induces pain. The patient's diminution of appetite is partly related to his avoidance of food out of fear of inducing abdominal pain. The patient's weight loss may be attributed to his decreased appetite and caloric intake as well as malabsorption caused by a reduction of pancreatic enzymes needed for the proper digestion and absorption of nutrients. The physical findings of abdominal tenderness relate to the patient's swollen pancreas. His decreased subcutaneous fat, temporal wasting, and sunken supraclavicular fossa are signs seen in malabsorption. The patient's decrease in pancreatic lipase and possible disturbance of his enterohepatic circulation are probable causes for his steatorrhea. You control the patient's pain, provide both nutritional support and pancreatic enzyme replacement, and advise him to stop drinking.

4.11 Answers to Reality Checks

Reality check 4-1: Parasympathetic stimulation of the salivary glands increases salivation. The administration of atropine, an anticholinergic medication, decreases salivary secretion and results in the patient's complaints of a dry mouth.

Reality check 4-2: The presence of a meal in the stomach stimulates the secretion of HCl into the gastric lumen and the subsequent absorption of HCO_3^- across the basolateral membrane of the parietal cell and into the gastric venous blood. The increase in HCO_3^- in the gastric venous blood raises the pH of the systemic blood and is referred to as the "alkaline tide." The absorbed HCO_3^- will eventually be secreted back into the GI tract via the pancreatic secretions.

Reality check 4-3: Cimetidine and other H_2 receptor blocking agents are very effective in treating peptic ulcers because they block both histamine stimulation at the H_2 receptor site of the parietal cell and the potentiating effects of histamine on gastrin and ACh.

Reality check 4-4: Gastric ulcer patients generally have decreased H^+ secretion because these patients experience a leak of H^+ back into and through the injured stomach mucosa. The reduction of H^+ secretion in gastric ulcer patients stimulates the G cells to secrete more gastrin.

Reality check 4-5: ACh is a neurotransmitter released from the vagus nerve that stimulates the M_3 receptor on the parietal cell to secrete H^+. Atropine is an anticholinergic or antimuscarinic agent which blocks the stimulation of ACh at the M_3 receptor which leads to a reduction of H^+ secretion. The paracrine, histamine, is released from gastric mucosal ECL cells and diffuses a short distance to the parietal cells. When histamine binds to the H_2 receptor, H^+ secretion is stimulated via the second messenger cAMP. Drugs such as cimetidine are called H_2 receptor blocking agents because they inhibit the secretion of H^+ due to histamines. The H^+–K^+ ATPase pump is located in the apical (luminal) side of the parietal cell and secretes H^+ into the gastric lumen. You could think of drugs like omeprazole (proton pump inhibitors) as "smart bombs" which inhibit the secretion of H^+ at the H^+–K^+ pumps and effectively take out the H^+ secreting factories.

Reality check 4-6: Patients with cystic fibrosis (CF) develop inspissated mucus in the pancreatic ducts which leads to ductal obstruction and pancreatic insufficiency. CF patients cannot produce an adequate amount of pancreatic enzymes needed to properly digest carbohydrates, proteins, and lipids. Therefore, CF patients develop malabsorption and diarrhea.

Reality check 4-7: Destruction of the absorptive surface area of the terminal ileum in the Crohn's disease patient results in an interruption of the enterohepatic circulation of bile salts and an increase in the excretion of bile salts in the stool. Because the fecal loss of bile salts exceeds the synthesis of new bile salts, there will be a reduction of the bile salt pool which will lead to lipid malabsorption and increased fat in the stool (steatorrhea).

Reality check 4-8: In the intestinal cell, the lipid products of digestion are reesterified with free fatty acids and combine with apoproteins to form chylomicrons which undergo exocytosis resulting in transport of lipids into the lymphatic circulation and ultimately into the blood. The absence of apoproteins results in the malabsorption of lipids. Hence, patients with abetalipoproteinemia will suffer from malabsorption of lipids and will have steatorrhea.

Reality check 4-9: The short bowel syndrome results from the surgical removal or bypassing greater than 50–60 % of the absorptive surface area of the small intestine, which is the major site of nutrient absorption. Long-term effects of the short bowel syndrome include weight loss, chronic diarrhea, and vitamin and mineral deficiencies, e.g., B vitamins including B12 and folate, as well as iron, calcium, zinc. In addition, the reduction of nutrients, vitamins, and minerals may result in anemia.

4.12   Answers to Review Questions

4-1. **A.** Saliva composition varies with the rate of salivary flow. At low flow rates, the salivary ducts will have an ample amount of time to reabsorb NaCl or secrete K^+. On the contrary, at high salivary flow rates, the salivary ducts will not have enough time to reabsorb NaCl or secrete K^+; hence, the saliva will resemble the initial saliva produced by the acinar cells.

4-2. **B.** The gastric parietal cells secrete intrinsic factor (the only essential component of gastric juice). Intrinsic factor forms a complex with vitamin B12 that is absorbed in the terminal ileum. Once a patient's stomach has been removed, then the patient cannot produce intrinsic factor which is needed for vitamin B12 absorption. In order to work around this absorption problem, the patient must receive vitamin B12 by injection because an oral form would be subject to protein digestion.

4-3. **D.** The primary function of secretin is to stimulate pancreatic bicarbonate secretion. Hence, if one administers IV secretin to a normal volunteer, one would expect to see an increase in pancreatic bicarbonate secretion. This is the basis of the IV secretin pancreatic function test. In patients with chronic pancreatitis and pancreatic insufficiency, one would expect to see a suboptimal production of bicarbonate secretion.

4-4. **A.** When the bile salt SGC (pK $= 2$) is present in the duodenal lumen (pK $= 3$–5), SGC will act as an acid and donate H^+, thus it will be in its ionized form (SGC$^-$) and will be more water soluble. Because bile salts are amphipathic (contain hydrophilic and hydrophobic sections), above a critical bile salt concentration, they will form micelles and transport cholesterol and the lipid products of digestion to the intestinal cell's brush border for absorption.

4-5. **D.** Remember to keep it straight. Na^+ absorption in the colon occurs primarily by passive diffusion. In the small intestine, NaCl absorption occurs primarily by cotransport mechanisms involving Na^+–glucose, Na^+–amino acid, or by Na^+–H^+ exchange.

Suggested Reading

Barrett KE. Gastric secretion (Chapter 50). In: Raff H, Levitzky I, editors. Medical physiology: a systems approach. New York: McGraw Hill; 2011.

Hall JE. Secretory functions of the alimentary tract (Chapter 64). In: Hall JE, editor. Guyton and Hall textbook of medical physiology. Philadelphia: Saunders Elsevier; 2011.

Janson LW, Tischler ME. The digestive system (Chapter 11). In: The big picture: medical biochemistry. New York: McGraw Hill; 2012. p. 149–66.

Johnson LR. Salivary secretion (Chapter 7). In: Gastrointestinal physiology. 8th ed. Philadelphia: Elsevier-Mosby; 2014a. p. 54–63.

Johnson LR. Pancreatic secretion (Chapter 9). In: Gastrointestinal physiology. 8th ed. Philadelphia: Elsevier-Mosby; 2014b. p. 82–93.

Johnson LR. Bile secretion and gallbladder function (Chapter 10). In: Gastrointestinal physiology. 8th ed. Philadelphia: Elsevier-Mosby; 2014c. p. 94–107.

Chapter 5
Physiology of the Liver, Gallbladder and Pancreas: "Getting By" with Some Help from Your Friends

5.1 Introduction

Lipids are necessary for many important processes in the body. Here we discuss how the digestion and absorption of lipids require the adequate synthesis of primary bile acids and bile salts and the circulation of the bile salts between the intestine and the liver (enterohepatic). Let us examine the function of the three cell types within the liver as well as the key biosynthetic pathways for bile acids and bile salts in order to better understand their roles in lipid digestion and absorption.

5.2 Liver

5.2.1 Function of the Three Main Cell Types Within the Liver

The three main cell types within the liver include *hepatocytes* (~75 % of the liver mass), sinusoidal lining cells (*Kupffer cells*, *stellate cells*, and *endothelial cells*), and cells that form the bile ducts.

Hepatocytes uniquely produce their own structural proteins and intracellular enzymes in addition to fibrinogen, prothrombin group clotting factors, and albumin. Hepatocytes also mainly produce transferrin, glycoproteins, lipoproteins, and ceruloplasmin. The rough endoplasmic reticulum, a hepatocyte organelle, is the site of protein synthesis. Once the proteins form, both the smooth reticulum and rough endoplasmic reticulum play a role in the secretion of the formed proteins. The endoplasmic reticulum also plays an important role in the conjugation of proteins to carbohydrate and lipid moieties modified or made in the hepatocytes.

Glucose homeostasis depends on hepatocyte functions. After food is absorbed in the small intestine, the portal system carries the primary dietary carbohydrates (i.e., glucose, fructose, and galactose) to the liver. After uptake by hepatocytes, these

E. Trowers and M. Tischler, *Gastrointestinal Physiology*,
DOI 10.1007/978-3-319-07164-0_5, © Springer International Publishing Switzerland 2014

carbohydrates are converted by cytosolic enzymes into phosphorylated sugars. Glucose replenishes the stores of *glycogen*, a glucose polymer. Galactose can be converted into phosphorylated glucose and also be stored as glycogen. Depending on the amount of glucose in the diet, fructose may be metabolized to glucose to maintain glucose homeostasis. In addition, hepatocytes serve as an important storage site for iron, vitamin B12, and vitamin A.

Fatty acids are formed in the liver from excess dietary carbohydrates. Glycerol and fatty acids combine to form triglycerides in the liver. Certain apoproteins are synthesized in the hepatocytes and are used in the assembly and export of lipoproteins (high density lipoprotein, HDL; very low density lipoprotein, VLDL). The liver synthesizes cholesterol from saturated fatty acids via acetate, in the form of acetyl CoA, and serves as the sole site for the formation of bile acids from cholesterol. Other important functions of the hepatocytes include the reception of many lipids from the systemic circulation and the metabolism of *chylomicron remnants* carrying dietary cholesterol and fat soluble vitamins.

The secretion of lipids into the bile is closely related to the metabolism of bile acids, lipoproteins, cholesterol, and phospholipids. The production of gallstones is associated with the biochemical alterations of bile.

Hepatocytes detoxify exogenous compounds (e.g., drugs or insecticides) and endogenous compounds (e.g., steroids). During Stage I reactions, the *cytochrome P450* enzymes are involved in metabolic transformations (e.g., hydroxylation or oxidation). Stage II reactions are characterized by the conjugation of Stage I metabolites with either glutathione or glucuronic acid in preparation for excretion. Steroid hormones and other compounds are converted into inactive forms. On the other hand, some compounds may be converted into more biologically functional forms via reactions in the hepatocytes.

A number of substances (e.g., drugs or bilirubin) are conjugated and converted into a more water soluble state in preparation for excretion via the bile. Thus, when patients with cirrhosis present with a severe decrease in liver function, they often encounter serious side effects from small amounts of drugs that cannot be detoxified or excreted. Bile duct cells create a tubular conduit for the passage of bile from the liver into the gut. These cells, under the influence of neurohumoral stimulation, alter the water and electrolyte composition of bile as it flows down the bile duct.

The sinusoids of the liver are lined by Kupffer cells, which are connected to endothelial cells. Kupffer cells, which are derived from monocytes, represent the largest group of fixed macrophages found in the body. These cells phagocytose bacteria, old cells, and tumor cells, and make the liver sinusoids a site for the clearance of particulate matter from the plasma. Hence, the liver plays a very important role as a filter.

Stellate cells, also known as Ito cells or lipocytes, resemble fibroblasts and are relatively small in size. These cells are characterized by having many droplets of fat in their cytoplasm. Stellate cells play an important role in fibrogenesis, which is a key pathological component of cirrhosis and chronic liver disease. Additionally, stellate cells store vitamin A as retinol palmitate.

5.3 Formation of Bile Acids and Salts

Bile, which is constantly produced by the hepatocytes, is primarily stored in the gallbladder. Approximately 450 mL of bile is secreted in 12 h. The maximum volume of the gallbladder is about 30–60 mL. Due to the continuous absorption of water, sodium, chloride, and other electrolytes, the bile salts, cholesterol, lecithin, and lipids, which are not reabsorbed, significantly increase their concentrations in the bile. Bile salts account for approximately half of the solutes in bile.

Bile consists of two key constituents, namely, *bile acids* and *bile salts*. The rate limiting enzyme 7α-hydroxylase converts cholesterol into 7α-hydroxycholesterol that is then metabolized into the primary bile acids cholic acid and chenodeoxycholic acid (Fig. 5.1). Increased production of cholic acid results in feedback inhibition of this biosynthetic pathway. Secondary bile acids (deoxycholic acid and lithocholic acid) result from the dehydroxylation of primary bile acids by bacteria when bile containing the primary bile acids is secreted into the intestinal lumen. Bile salts form when bile acids conjugate with either taurine or glycine. Conjugation of taurine with cholic acid results in taurocholic acid. There are a total of eight possible bile salts. By conjugating bile acids to form bile salts, the pK_a of the molecule decreases making the bile salts more soluble in the aqueous environment of the intestinal lumen. Consider that the pH of duodenal contents generally is in the range of 3–5. Because bile acids have a pK_a of ~7 they are almost always fully protonated in their nonionized form and hence are relatively water insoluble. In comparison the pK_a of bile salts ranges from 1 to 4. Consequently, bile salts exist primarily in their ionized form (A^-) and thus are water soluble.

Reality check 5-1: Patients with Zollinger–Ellison syndrome secrete massive amounts of gastric acid, which enters into their intestinal lumen. How does the decreased luminal pH affect the role of bile salts' in lipid absorption?

5.3.1 Recall Points

Key Processes in Bile Acid/Salt Formation and Action
- Cholesterol conversion into bile acids in the liver.
- Bile acid conjugation with taurine or glycine produces bile salts.
- Bile salts exhibit enhanced water solubility in the duodenum.

5.4 Lipid Absorption

When fatty foods enter the duodenum from the stomach, cholecystokinin (CCK) is released from I cells. CCK stimulates the gallbladder to contract and the sphincter of Oddi to relax (Fig. 5.2). This chain of events occurs about 30 min after a meal

Fig. 5.1 Biosynthesis of bile acids and bile salts

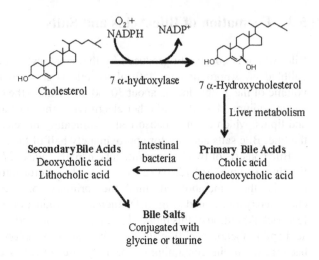

and results in the gallbladder emptying its store of bile into the duodenum to promote the digestion and absorption of lipids.

5.4.1 Emulsification

Why are bile salts so efficacious in lipid digestion and absorption? Bile salts are amphipathic molecules because they contain both a hydrophilic and a hydrophobic portion. The hydrophilic portion of a bile salt is negatively charged and points outward from the hydrophobic center. Therefore, the hydrophilic portion of a bile salt dissolves in the aqueous phase and the hydrophobic portion dissolves in the lipid phase. In an aqueous environment, bile salts arrange themselves around lipids with the negatively charged hydrophilic portion repelling similarly charged neighboring bile salt/lipid pairings. Thus the lipids disperse into small droplets via a process called *emulsification*. The stomach also plays an important role in emulsification when it mechanically agitates foodstuffs. In the gastrointestinal lumen, emulsification results in an increase of lipid's contact area with water and increases the water–oil interface where lipid digestive enzymes can work.

5.4.2 Micelle Formation

The pancreatic lipases (*pancreatic lipase, phospholipase A2*, and *cholesterol esterase*) hydrolyze lipids to the lipid breakdown products (free fatty acids, monoglycerides, lysolecithin, and cholesterol). These lipid breakdown products are solubilized in the intestinal lumen via micelles (Fig. 5.2; see also Fig. 4.7).

Fig. 5.2 Effect of cholecystokinin on gallbladder contraction {**C**} and sphincter of Oddi relaxation {**R**}, and the recycling of bile salts. *CCK* cholecystokinin, *FFA* free fatty acids

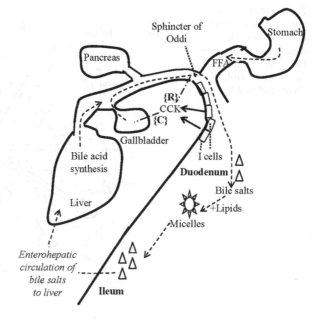

The center of the micelle contains the lipid digestion products and the external portion is lined with amphipathic bile salts (Fig. 5.3). Hence, the hydrophilic portion of the bile salts will be dissolved in the aqueous portion of the intestinal lumen, while the lipids will be solubilized in the micelle core. Because the micelle's outer surface is water soluble, it can interact with the intestinal cell's brush border. Once the micelle contacts the brush border, the lipid products of digestion freely diffuse into the interior of the intestinal cell through the luminal plasma membrane (see Fig. 4.8). The bile salts do not enter into the intestinal cell and remain in the intestinal lumen to form new micelles with new lipid products of digestion. A critical mass of bile salts is required for the formation of micelles. Once inside the intestinal cell, the lipid digestion products are reesterified to triglycerides, phospholipids, and cholesterol ester, which in turn are combined with Apoprotein B to form *chylomicrons*. The intestinal cell plasma membrane fuses with the chylomicron and extrudes it into the lymph vessels via exocytosis because the chylomicrons are too large to directly enter the surrounding capillaries and blood. Abetalipoproteinemia is a disorder in which patients lack Apoprotein B or microsomal triglyceride transfer protein and consequently cannot transport chylomicrons out of the intestinal cell leading to problems with lipid absorption.

Reality check 5-2: A patient with hyperlipidemia (increased lipids in the blood) was prescribed cholestyramine (a bile salt binding agent) and a low fat diet. Why?

Case in Point 5-1

Fig. 5.3 Structure of micelles. Micelles emulsify the products of lipid digestion including free fatty acid, monoacylglycerol, cholesterol, and lysolecithin

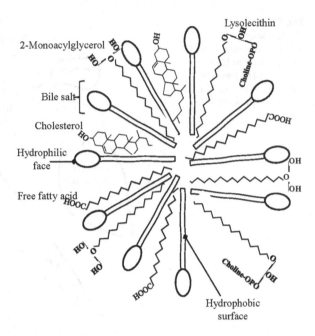

Chief Complaint: Unexplained weight loss, diarrhea, vomiting, and weakness in the extremities

History: A 52-year-old Caucasian man presents with diarrhea, vomiting, fatty, foul-smelling stools, and weight loss of 22 lb over the last 2 months. He reports abdominal pain that is usually more severe after eating. He reports weakness in the extremities as well as joint pain over the past year but has simply taken ibuprofen to treat the symptoms. He also reports that lately he has been having trouble recalling small details.

Physical Exam: A middle-aged man appearing chronically ill and in moderate distress. Vital signs are temperature 99.6 °F, blood pressure 110/70 mmHg, pulse 110/min, and respirations 17/min. Physical examination shows diffuse hyperpigmentation, leg edema, pleural effusion, and joint pain with symptoms of arthritis.

Labs:

Hb 10.3 g/dL [*N*: 13.8–17.2]	Hct 31 % [*N*: 41–52 %]
RBC 4.1 × 10^6 cells/μL [*N*: 4.4–5.8]	WBC 15.1 × 10^3 cells/μL [*N*: 3.8–10.8]
Neutrophils 9,500 cells/μL [*N*: 1,500–7,800]	Platelets 500 × 10^9 cells/L [*N*: 150–450]
MCV 75.6 fL [*N*: 80–100] [microcytosis]	MCH 25.1 pg [*N*: 27–31] [hypochromia]
Prothrombin time 10 s [*N*: 9–12.5]	
Sodium 149 mEq/L [*N*: 135–147]	Potassium 3.5 mEq/L [*N*: 3.5–5.2]
Chloride 94 mEq/L [*N*: 95–107]	Bicarbonate 20 mM [*N*: 22–29]
Creatinine 0.9 mg/dL [normal 0.7–1.2]	Alkaline phosphatase 350 U/L [*N*: <120]
Albumin 2.8 g/dL [*N*: 3.5–5]	Folic acid 2.1 ng/mL [*N*: >1.9]
Vitamin A 25 μg/dL [*N*: 30–95]	Vitamin B12:300 pg/mL [*N*: 200–800]

(continued)

Vitamin E 3 µg/mL [*N*: 5–20]	Iron 18 µg/dL [*N*: 25–170]
γ-Glutamyl transpeptidase 125 U/L [*N*: <65]	

Assessment: On the basis of these findings, (1) what is the likely diagnosis for this patient; (2) why does the patient have anemia with microcytosis and hypochromia; (3) what is the likely reason for the neurological symptoms; and (4) why does the patient have edema?

5.5 Enterohepatic Circulation

Once lipid absorption is complete, the bile salts are absorbed from the terminal ileum into the portal circulation by Na^+-bile salt cotransporters and are extracted by the hepatocytes. During this *enterohepatic circulation* process the great majority of bile salts are recirculated (Fig. 5.2). Therefore, there is a reduced need for the synthesis of new bile salts. The frugal liver needs only to replace the small amount of bile salts lost in the feces.

5.5.1 Recall Points

Enterohepatic Circulation
- CCK stimulates gallbladder contraction and sphincter of Oddi relaxation.
- Micelles transport lipid breakdown products to intestinal epithelial cells.
- Enterohepatic circulation preserves bile salt pool.

Reality check 5-3: Patients with Crohn's disease (an inflammatory bowel disease characterized by transmural thickening of the intestinal wall frequently involving the terminal ileum) may present with steatorrhea. Why?

5.6 Bile Pigment Processing

As noted above, besides bile salts, conjugated bilirubin is also excreted via the bile. Bilirubin is made from breakdown of the heme porphyrin ring when red cells are lysed (Fig. 5.4). This form of bilirubin is water insoluble and therefore cannot be excreted in the urine. Excessive hemolysis thus increases the circulating amount of unconjugated bilirubin leading to one cause of *jaundice*. To be excreted, bilirubin

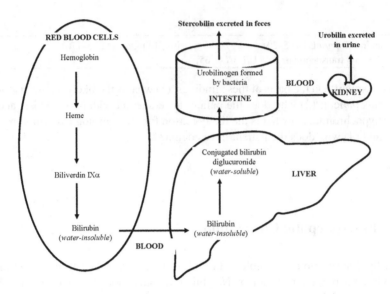

Fig. 5.4 Synthesis and processing of bilirubin. Bilirubin derived heme is conjugated in the liver to a soluble form that can be excreted in the bile. Intestinal bacteria process conjugated bilirubin to urobilinogen that is either excreted in the feces as stercobilin or absorbed into the blood for excretion in the urine as urobilin. *UDPG* UDP-glucuronic acid

must be conjugated with glucuronic acid in a hepatic reaction catalyzed by *UDP-glucuronyltransferase* and then excreted in the bile.

There are two syndromes in which conjugation of bilirubin is impaired due to lower activity of the UDP-glucuronyltransferase. *Gilbert's syndrome* is a milder disease because significant activity of the enzyme remains. Hence these patients exhibit a mild increase in unconjugated bilirubin. In contrast, *Crigler–Najjar syndrome* is caused by a severely defective enzyme resulting in a marked increase of circulating unconjugated bilirubin. *Hepatitis* causes a *mixed hyperbilirubinemia* because less unconjugated bilirubin can be conjugated and of the amount conjugated not all of it can be excreted. Hence patients with hepatitis or other liver damage exhibit jaundice associated with both forms of bilirubin elevated in the blood and conjugated bilirubin appearing in the urine. Patients with *Dubin–Johnson syndrome* have diminished transport of conjugated bilirubin into the biliary system and hence exhibit elevated conjugated bilirubin in both the blood and urine.

Once conjugated bilirubin enters the intestine, gut bacteria convert it into urobilinogen. Urobilinogen is then either oxidized to stercobilin for excretion in the feces (providing the dark color) or absorbed in the ileum. Once urobilinogen enters the blood it is excreted in the urine where it is oxidized to urobilin (yellow color of the urine).

5.6.1 Recall Points

Bile Pigment Processing
- Bilirubin is produced from heme breakdown.
- Conjugated bilirubin is produced in the liver for excretion.

5.7 Pancreatic Exocrine Secretion

The pancreas has both an exocrine (90 %) portion and an endocrine (10 %) portion. The exocrine cells of the pancreas produce secretions that flow out of the body of the gland via a duct. Similar to the salivary glands, the exocrine pancreas is composed of *acini*, which are small collections of serous cells arranged around a secretory duct (see Fig. 4.6). In addition, the exocrine portion of the pancreas produces an enzymatic secretion via the acinar cells and an aqueous component secreted by the centroacinar cells and subsequently modified by the ductal cells. On the other hand, the endocrine function of the pancreas is mediated via the action of hormones.

Most of the enzymes required for the digestion of a mixed meal (foodstuff consisting of carbohydrates, proteins, or fats in any combination) are produced by the exocrine pancreas. For impairment of the digestion of fat to occur, pancreas secretion must be reduced to less than 10 % of its normal output or the flow of pancreatic juice into the intestine becomes physically obstructed.

Pancreatic digestive enzymes include several hydrolytic pancreatic lipases (pancreatic lipase, cholesterol esterase, phospholipase A_2), amylase, and a variety of proteases. Amylase and cholesterol esterase are secreted in active forms but not so for the other digestive enzymes. Pancreatic lipase activity requires colipase, which is also secreted by the pancreas but in an inactive procolipase form that is activated by trypsin. Similarly phospholipase A_2 is activated by trypsin from its inactive pro-phospholipase A_2 form. Pancreatic proteases are also secreted in inactive forms into the duodenal lumen where they are activated by trypsin, which itself is initially activated from trypsinogen by enteropeptidase that is secreted by duodenal cells. Trypsin can then activate additional molecules of trypsinogen. Pancreatic digestive enzymes are synthesized in the rough endoplasmic reticulum of the pancreatic acinar cells. Next, the newly synthesized digestive enzymes are transferred to the Golgi complex for concentration into zymogen granules, which will be released upon the arrival of a stimulus, e.g., CCK and parasympathetic activity.

The aqueous portion of pancreatic secretion is an ultrafiltrate of plasma that is secondarily modified in the duct. Initially, an isotonic solution is produced by the centroacinar and ductal cells that contains bicarbonate, sodium, potassium, and chloride concentrations. The ductal cells change the composition of the initial pancreatic secretion by the secretion of bicarbonate and the absorption of Cl^- via a luminal membrane Cl^-–HCO_3^- exchange apparatus.

That pancreatic secretions vary with flow rate is a critically important concept to keep in mind. A change in the rate of flow of the pancreatic juice causes the concentrations of HCO_3^- and Cl^- to change, whereas Na^+ and K^+ concentrations remain constant. At low flow rates, an isotonic solution of pancreatic juice contains primarily Na^+, Cl^-, and water. Stimulation of the centroacinar and ductal cells via an agent, e.g., secretin, causes a greater amount of an isotonic solution to be produced with a composition of Na^+, HCO_3^-, and water. There are two theories to explain the flow-related composition of pancreatic juice.

The two-component theory assumes that the acinar cell secretes a small amount of fluid, which contains primarily Na^+ and Cl^-. The duct cells secrete large volumes of pancreatic juice containing primarily Na^+ and HCO_3^- in response to stimulation. Hence, when the rate of secretion is low, the relative concentration of Cl^- will be high. At high secretory rates, the fixed amount of Cl^- being secreted will be diluted by the larger volume of HCO_3^- containing juice.

An alternate theory proposes that the cells primarily secrete HCO_3^- and that as the pancreatic juice moves down the ducts HCO_3^- and Cl^- are exchanged. At low pancreatic juice flow rates there is ample time for Cl^- and HCO_3^- exchange and the concentration of both anions then will be equal to their concentration in the plasma. However, at high pancreatic juice flow rates, there is less time for exchange and pancreatic juice will contain primarily HCO_3^- and Na^+.

5.7.1 Stimulation of Pancreatic Exocrine Secretion

The presence of H^+ in the duodenal lumen triggers the secretion by the duodenal S cells of secretin, which can then stimulate duct cells of both liver and pancreas. Secretin, acting via cAMP, stimulates the ductal cells to increase bicarbonate secretion in order to neutralize the luminal H^+ (Fig. 5.5). This HCO_3^- secretion is accomplished as follows. Cyclic AMP-dependent protein kinase A phosphorylates and thereby opens the CFTR channel allowing secretion of Cl^-. Intracellular carbonic anhydrase facilitates the combination of H_2O and CO_2 to produce H_2CO_3 which separates into HCO_3^- and H^+. The Cl^-–HCO_3^- exchanger found in the apical membrane of the ductal cell then secretes HCO_3^- into the pancreatic juice. The Na^+–H^+ exchanger located in the basolateral membrane of the ductal cell transports H^+ into the blood. The final result is a net secretion of bicarbonate into the pancreatic duct and a net absorption of H^+.

Reality check 5-4: Endoscopic retrograde cholangiopancreatography (ERCP) is a procedure in which an endoscopist passes an endoscope through the mouth, esophagus, and stomach and then into the duodenum. Once the papilla is found it is cannulated and dye is injected into the pancreatic duct to produce an x-ray image. Patients with pancreas divisum have a minor and major pancreatic duct. Occasionally, when the endoscopists cannot locate the minor papilla and minor pancreatic duct, they give the patient an intravenous injection of secretin. Why?

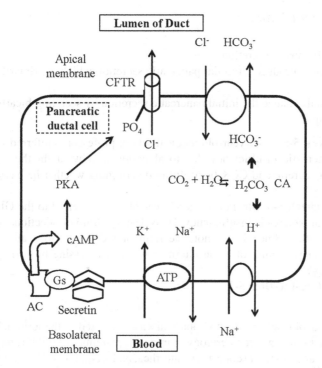

Fig. 5.5 Secretion of bicarbonate by pancreatic ductal cells in response to secretin. Secretin binds to its receptor, which interacts with Gs protein that in turn activates adenylyl cyclase (AC) to produce cAMP. The cAMP-dependent protein kinase A (PKA) opens the chloride channel (CFTR) allowing secretion of Cl⁻. Bicarbonate, which is produced by the action of carbonic anhydrase (CA), undergoes exchange transport with this Cl⁻ and once secreted neutralizes acid in the pancreatic duct. The H⁺ produced by the same CA reaction is secreted to the blood in exchange for Na⁺ that is itself secreted in exchange for K⁺ via the Na⁺–K⁺ pump (ATP)

The presence of fatty acids, amino acids, and small peptides in the duodenal lumen triggers the secretion of CCK by the duodenal I cells (Fig. 5.2). CCK stimulates the acinar cells to raise their secretion of the digestive enzymes, lipase, protease and amylase. CCK potentiates the effect of secretin on the pancreatic ductal cells and stimulates the secretion of bicarbonate because of the different mechanisms of action of IP$_3$ and increased intracellular [Ca^{2+}] (the second messengers for CCK), whereas cAMP is the second messenger for secretin. Fatty acids, H$^+$, small peptides, and amino acids when present in the duodenal lumen stimulate the release of acetylcholine via vagovagal reflexes.

Patients who have sustained approximately 90 % damage to the exocrine portion of their pancreas, whether due to chronic pancreatitis or disorder of pancreatic secretion such as cystic fibrosis, will be unable to produce a sufficient amount of pancreatic enzymes and will suffer from malabsorption.

5.7.2 Recall Points

Pancreatic Exocrine Secretion
- Acinar cells produce an initial pancreatic secretion which is primarily Na^+ and Cl^-.
- Ductal cells change the initial pancreatic secretion by secreting bicarbonate and absorbing Cl^-.

Reality check 5-5: A 45-year-old medical school professor is referred for evaluation of pancreatic insufficiency due to alcoholism. Why might the intravenous injection of secretin and CCK be useful in determining whether he has pancreatic insufficiency?

Reality check 5-6: Mr. Pollo is a 57-year-old man referred to the GI clinic for evaluation of pancreatic insufficiency. He is deathly afraid of injections or even the sight of needles. Since intravenous secretin or CCK injections are out of the question, can you think of some alternate ways of assessing him for pancreatic insufficiency?

Connecting-the-Dots 5-1

A 37-year-old woman with Crohn's disease localized to the terminal ileum presents to the gastroenterology clinic complaining of mild right lower quadrant abdominal discomfort, steatorrhea, and weight loss. Crohn's disease is an inflammatory bowel disease characterized by transmural thickening of the intestinal wall. On physical examination, she appears chronically ill, but in no acute distress. The respiratory rate is 14/min, and her breath sounds are clear to auscultation. The abdominal exam is remarkable for mild tenderness to deep palpation in the right lower quadrant and a mass the size of a small sausage. Laboratory findings were remarkable for a macrocytic anemia, fecal occult blood positivity, and increased fecal fat. In addition, abdominal CT scan shows thickening of the wall of the terminal ileum without signs of obstruction. What is the likely physiological cause of the patient's findings?

5.8 Summary Points

- Hepatocytes continuously produce bile that is stored in the gallbladder.
- Major constituents of bile include bile salts, cholesterol, lipids, lecithin, water, sodium, chloride, and other electrolytes.
- The rate limiting enzyme in the conversion of cholesterol to bile acids is 7α-hydroxylase.
- Cholic acid and chenodeoxycholic acid are the primary bile acids.

- Secondary bile acids, deoxycholic acid, and lithocholic acid are produced by the action of intestinal bacteria on primary bile acids.
- Bile salts are produced by conjugation of bile acids with taurine or glycine.
- Bile salts have a decreased pK_a compared to bile acids and at the pH of the duodenal lumen bile salts, unlike bile acids, assume an ionized and more water soluble form.
- CCK is released from the duodenal I cells in the presence of fatty foods.
- CCK stimulates the gallbladder to contract and the sphincter of Oddi to relax.
- Bile salts are amphipathic. The hydrophilic portion dissolves in the aqueous phase and the hydrophobic portion dissolves in the lipid phase.
- Emulsification occurs when the negatively charged hydrophilic portions of bile salts repel neighboring negatively charged bile salts causing lipids to disperse into small droplets.
- Pancreatic lipases hydrolyze lipids to produce free fatty acids, monoacylglycerol, lysolecithin, and cholesterol.
- Mixed micelles solubilize lipid breakdown products in the intestinal lumen.
- The external portion of micelles is lined with amphipathic bile salts, and the center contains the lipid products of digestion.
- Lipid products of digestion diffuse into the interior of the intestinal cell while the bile salts remain in the lumen to form new micelles and ultimately to undergo enterohepatic circulation.
- Enterohepatic circulation occurs when bile salts are absorbed from the terminal ileum into the circulation by Na^+-bile salt cotransporters and extracted by the liver cells.
- Unconjugated bilirubin produced from heme breakdown cannot be excreted because it is not water soluble.
- Bilirubin is solubilized to a conjugated form in the liver and processed further in the intestine for excretion as stercobilin.
- Some urobilinogen is absorbed and excreted as urobilin in the urine.
- Chylomicrons form inside intestinal cells via the combination of Apoprotein B, triglycerides, phospholipids, and cholesterol ester.
- Chylomicrons undergo exocytosis into the lymph vessels.
- The exocrine pancreas secretion has a concentration high in bicarbonate, with sodium and potassium concentration similar to the plasma.
- Pancreatic acinar cells produce an initial secretion which is primarily Na^+ and Cl^-.
- Pancreatic ductal cells are responsible for the secretion of bicarbonate and the absorption of chloride.
- Intestinal S cells secrete secretin, which stimulates duct cells of both liver and pancreas.
- Secretion of CCK is stimulated by the duodenal I cells in response to the presence of fatty acids, amino acids, and small peptides.

5.9 Review Questions

5-1. You are taking care of a patient in the surgery clinic who has had a cholecystectomy (gallbladder removal). Which of the following offers the best physiological explanation for this patient's ability to digest lipids?

    A. Enterohepatic circulation is interrupted
    B. Gallbladder is not required for bile storage
    C. Gallbladder plays no role in lipid digestion
    D. Hepatocytes continuously produce bile

5-2. A patient with Zollinger–Ellison syndrome exhibits a markedly lower intraduodenal pH. Which of the following explains why this patient presents with steatorrhea?

    A. Bile salts will be in a nonionized form and will be absorbed prematurely by intestinal cells
    B. Bile salts will be in a nonionized form and will not be absorbed
    C. Bile salts will be in an ionized form and will be absorbed prematurely by the intestinal cells
    D. Bile salts will be in an ionized form and will not be absorbed

5-3. A start-up company is contemplating the production of the most potent proton pump inhibitor in order to corner the multibillion dollar antacid market. Assuming that this wonder drug virtually eliminates the presence of H^+ in the duodenal lumen, what effect would you expect concerning bicarbonate secretion by the pancreatic ductal cells?

    A. Decreased secretion
    B. Increased secretion
    C. No change in secretion

5-4. Let us assume that you are able to perform a microassay of pancreatic secretion at the level of the acinar cells prior to its entry into the pancreatic ductal cells. What would you expect to find in your sample of the initial pancreatic acinar secretion?

    A. Increased concentration of bicarbonate but decreased concentration of chloride
    B. Increased concentration of bicarbonate but decreased concentration of sodium
    C. Increased concentration of both bicarbonate and chloride
    D. Increased concentration of both sodium and chloride

5-5. You are in the surgery recovery room after completing a 50 % pancreatic resection on a patient who had received a gunshot wound to the abdomen. The patient wants to know if he can expect to develop malabsorption due to the removal of half of his pancreas. Based upon your understanding of the physiology of the exocrine pancreas, how would you respond to the patient?

A. Will develop malabsorption due to pancreatic insufficiency
B. Will not be expected to survive
C. Will probably not develop malabsorption due to pancreatic insufficiency

5.10 Answer to Case in Point

Case in Point 5-1: The patient shows many of the classic symptoms of a fat malabsorption malady. What is unique amongst the patient's symptoms, relative to more common fat digestion or malabsorption diseases are the diffuse hyperpigmentation, joint pain, and recent memory problem. The patient has Whipple's disease which is a rare bacterial infection caused by *Tropheryma whipplei*. Associated with the systemic infection is leukocytosis (elevated white blood cells), mild neutrophilia, and mild thrombocytosis (elevated platelet count). The fat malabsorption issues result from fat deposit (chylomicrons) blockage of the lymphatics associated with intestinal enterocytes. This interruption of chylomicron translocation backs up absorption, so that both mucosal and lymphatic diseases lead to steatorrhea and diarrhea. Besides the chronic diarrhea due to steatorrhea, patients classically exhibit joint pain, weight loss (due to malabsorption), abdominal pain/bloating, fatigue, and anemia. The anemia is primarily associated with iron deficiency due to malabsorption and as evidenced by the hypochromia and microcytosis. In contrast deficiencies of folate or vitamin B12 lead to hyperchromic, macrocytic anemia. Malabsorption of fat soluble vitamins in particular will cause some of the secondary symptoms. In this patient vitamin E deficiency would cause his neurological symptoms. Liver damage, as indicated by elevated gamma-glutamyl transpeptidase and to some extent the alkaline phosphatase, likely caused the hypoalbuminemia, which in turn caused peripheral edema in the patient.

The infection may be associated with a defective immune response and consequently patients can present with arthritis and joint pain related to this problem. This disease is most commonly found in middle-aged Caucasian men. Diagnosis can include use of endoscopy of the small intestine lining with a biopsy taken. Confirmation of the disease is best obtained by PCR testing for the bacterium or electron microscopy, which can identify these organisms because of their unique appearance. Because this lipid disorder is a secondary consequence of the infection, treatment is with antibiotics. This treatment is done for a year to be sure the bacteria are completely destroyed since shorter treatments may lead to a relapse. Symptoms subside within a week of initiating treatment barring the prior development of serious complications involving the brain and/or nervous system.

5.11 Answer to Connecting-the-Dots

Connecting-the-Dots 5-1: The terminal ileum generally resides in the right lower abdominal quadrant. A thickened intestinal wall in this region is the most probable cause of the small sausage size mass and mild discomfort to deep palpation in the area. Patients with transmural thickening of their terminal ileum will have a disruption of the enterohepatic circulation. This thickening will result in the malabsorption of lipids and causes steatorrhea. In addition, the terminal ileum is the site of vitamin B12 absorption. A deficiency of vitamin B12 results in an impairment of red blood cell metabolism manifested as a macrocytic (enlarged cell), hyperchromic anemia. The function of the terminal ileum may be restored via treatment with anti-inflammatory and immunosuppressive medications.

5.12 Answers to Reality Checks

Reality check 5-1: Bile salts are weak acids. In the presence of high acidity in the lumen of Zollinger–Ellison patients, bile salts will be in their nonionized (lipid soluble) form and will be absorbed prematurely in the small intestine. Hence, there will be a reduction in the amount of bile salts available for micelle formation and the absorption of lipids.

Reality check 5-2: Cholestyramine is a bile salt binding agent that will reduce the concentration of intraluminal bile salts needed for the absorption of lipids. Coupled with a low fat diet, bile salt binding agents reduce the amount of lipids absorbed from the intestinal lumen into the blood and are an effective treatment for increased lipids in the blood (hyperlipidemia).

Reality check 5-3: Crohn's disease patients with compromise of the absorptive surface area of the terminal ileum will experience an interruption of the enterohepatic circulation of bile salts. These patients will not have a sufficient amount of bile salts to form micelles and will not be able to absorb lipids effectively. Hence, they will present with steatorrhea.

Reality check 5-4: Secretin stimulates the secretion of pancreatic juice from the pancreatic duct. If the endoscopist gives a pancreas divisum patient intravenous secretin, then when the pancreatic juice exists from the minor papilla, they will observe its location.

Reality check 5-5: Intravenous secretin stimulates the pancreas to secrete bicarbonate that is important in creating a favorable intraluminal environment for digestive enzymes to work. Intravenous CCK stimulates the pancreas to secrete the digestive enzymes. A substandard response to the injection of secretin and CCK would be expected in a patient with pancreatic insufficiency.

Reality check 5-6: A Lundh test meal (containing protein, fat, and carbohydrates) would stimulate the pancreas to stimulate bicarbonate and digestive enzymes. A poor response to a Lundh test meal would be compatible with pancreatic insufficiency. Another approach would be to check his stools for increased fat due to malabsorption of lipids or a decreased level of a pancreatic protease such as fecal elastase.

5.13 Answers to Review Questions

5-1. **D.** Hepatocytes continuously produce bile. Hence, bile salts will be secreted into intestinal lumen for the absorption of lipids despite the absence of a gallbladder.

5-2. **A.** Bile salts have a pK of 1–4. If the duodenal lumen is markedly acidic, then the bile salts will be in their nonionized form and will be prematurely absorbed by the intestinal cells. Therefore, there will not be an adequate amount of bile salts for the absorption of lipids and the patient will present with steatorrhea. In addition, pancreatic lipases will be inactivated at an acidic pH.

5-3. **A.** The presence of H^+ in the duodenal lumen triggers the secretion of secretin by the S cells which results in an increase in bicarbonate secretion in order to neutralize the luminal H^+. If the amount of H^+ present in the duodenal lumen is markedly decreased, then the stimulus for bicarbonate secretion is reduced and one would expect a decrease in the secretion of bicarbonate by the pancreatic ductal cells.

5-4. **D.** Acinar cells produce an initial pancreatic secretion which is primarily Na^+ and Cl^-. Hence, a microassay at this level would reflect this finding. The ductal cells change the composition of the initial pancreatic secretion by the secretion of bicarbonate and the absorption of Cl^-.

5-5. **C.** Patients who suffer approximately 90 % damage to their pancreas will not be able to produce a sufficient amount of pancreatic enzymes and will develop malabsorption. However patients with half of their pancreas still functioning likely will produce and secrete sufficient digestive enzymes for digestion and absorption.

Suggested Reading

Janson LW, Tischler ME. The digestive system (Chapter 11). In: The big picture: medical biochemistry. New York: McGraw Hill; 2012. p. 149–66.

Johnson LR. Bile secretion and gallbladder function (Chapter 10). In: Gastrointestinal physiology. 8th ed. Philadelphia: Elsevier-Mosby; 2014. p. 94–107.

Kibble JD, Halsey CR. Gastrointestinal physiology (Chapter 7). In: The big picture: medical physiology. New York: McGraw Hill; 2009. p. 259–306.

Chapter 6
Nutrient Exchange: Matching Digestion and Absorption

6.1 Introduction

Having considered the physiological function of gastrointestinal secretions, we now consider details of the processes of digestion and absorption. How does the system get the products of digestion from the lumen, across the digestive tract cells, and into the blood? What are the effects of motility on digestion and absorption? What roles do gastrointestinal hormones play in digestion and absorption? These are just a few of the questions to be addressed.

6.2 Anatomy

The study of digestion and absorption begins by considering the relevant functional anatomy. Then we will turn our attention to the brain–gut axis' role and the interaction of digestion-related molecules which either directly attack carbohydrates, proteins, and lipids or work through cell-regulatory effects. Digestion and absorption require nutrient exchange. The correlation of these functions, or the lack thereof, determines whether we succeed or fail to thrive.

6.3 Digestion

During *digestion* food is physically broken up, through the action of the teeth or chemically through the action of enzymes, and changed into a substance appropriate for absorption and assimilation into the body or excretion from the body. In higher vertebrates and humans, digestion mainly occurs in the small intestine. *Absorption* involves the uptake of substances by a tissue, such as nutrients across the wall of the intestine. The salivary, gastric, pancreatic juices, and apical

E. Trowers and M. Tischler, *Gastrointestinal Physiology*,
DOI 10.1007/978-3-319-07164-0_6, © Springer International Publishing Switzerland 2014

membrane of the intestinal epithelial cells contain the enzymes involved in the process of digestion. Different digestive enzymes found at various locations along the gastrointestinal tract are involved in processing of the three major types of food—carbohydrates, lipids, and protein. However, hydrolysis, or the process in which substrate-specific enzymes lead to the breakdown of a macromolecule by the addition of water, is the main chemical process involved in the digestion of all major nutrients. In the ensuing sections, we will examine the major nutrient groups and their digestion and absorption.

6.3.1   Recall Points

Digestion
- Involves mechanical and chemical processes.
- Occurs mainly in the small intestine.
- Salivary, gastric, pancreatic juices as well as apical membrane of the intestinal cells contain digestive enzymes.
- Hydrolysis is the main chemical process of digestion.

6.3.2   Digestion of Carbohydrates

Most of the dietary carbohydrates are large polysaccharides (i.e., amylose or amylopectin) or disaccharides (i.e., lactose, sucrose, maltose, or trehalose), which represent monosaccharide groups bound together (Fig. 6.1). Carbohydrates must be broken down to the monosaccharides (glucose, galactose, and fructose) in order for absorption to take place.

The carbohydrate digestive enzyme, *amylase*, is found in both the saliva and pancreas. The digestion of carbohydrate polysaccharides begins with the action of alpha-amylase in the mouth but mostly the pancreatic amylase is responsible for the hydrolysis of the starches amylose and amylopectin. Amylase hydrolyzes starch by cleaving α1,4 glycosidic bonds, to smaller units including maltose, maltotriose, and oligosaccharides (up to nine glucose units) that are either branched (α-limit dextrin) or unbranched (Fig. 6.2).

The intestinal mucosa serves as the source of the other carbohydrate digestive enzymes. The intestinal brush border enzymes include four different complexes (Fig. 6.3). The *glucoamylase complex*, most often called *maltase*, catalyzes the hydrolysis of α1,4 glycosidic bonds in oligosaccharides to produce glucose, maltose, maltotriose, or isomaltose as products. Isomaltose contains an α1,6 glycosidic bond that is hydrolyzed to yield two glucose molecules by the action of *isomaltase* (also known as α-dextrinase or debranching enzyme) of the *sucrose–isomaltase complex*. The isomaltase also catalyzes the digestion of maltose and maltotriose to two and three glucose molecules, respectively, while sucrase hydrolyzes sucrose to

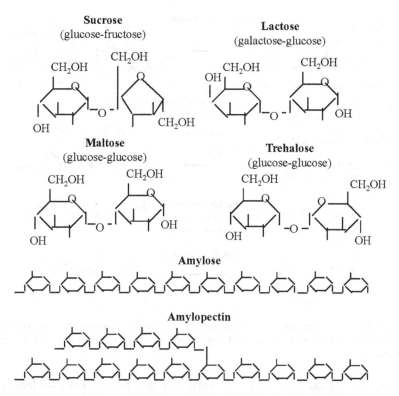

Fig. 6.1 The primary dietary carbohydrates. These include disaccharides as well as branched and unbranched plant glucose polymers, amylopectin, and amylose, respectively

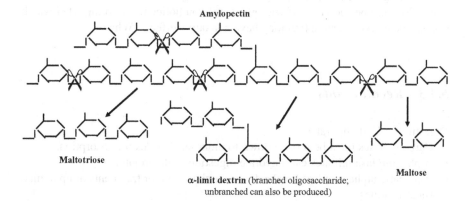

Fig. 6.2 Catalytic action of salivary or pancreatic amylase. Primary products include maltose, maltotriose, and oligosaccharides, for which the branched form is termed α-limit dextrin

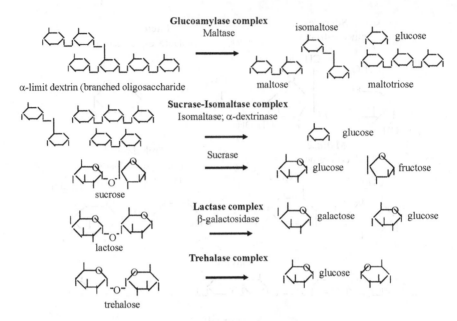

Fig. 6.3 Brush border carbohydrate digestive enzyme complexes. Complexes located in the small intestine brush border process products of amylose and amylopectin digestion as well as dietary disaccharides

fructose and glucose. *Lactase* (also known as *β-galactosidase*) cleaves lactose to glucose and galactose. *Trehalase* hydrolyzes trehalose to two glucose molecules.

Reality check 6-1: It is late at night and you have a craving for chocolates. As you rummage through the fridge, you notice a bag of delectable sugar-free chocolates. You are beside yourself with glee until you notice the warning label which states: "excessive consumption may have a laxative effect." Why?

6.3.3   *Recall Points*

Digestion of Carbohydrates
- Carbohydrates must be broken down to monosaccharides for absorption.
- Alpha-amylase initiates carbohydrate digestion in the mouth.
- Pancreatic alpha-amylase breaks down starch to smaller fragments of up to nine sugar residues.
- Intestinal brush border enzymes digest oligosaccharides, trisaccharides, and disaccharides to glucose, fructose, and galactose.

6.3.4   Digestion of Proteins

Proteins are created from amino acids joined by peptide linkages. Proteolytic enzymes split (hydrolyze) proteins and return them to their constituent amino acids via the addition of water molecules. The stomach is the source for the digestive enzyme *pepsin*. It is important to note that pepsin is not absolutely essential for protein digestion. The chief cells of the stomach secrete its inactive precursor, *pepsinogen*. The acidic gastric pH (optimum range 1–3) permits *autoactivation* that converts pepsinogen into the active enzyme pepsin, which in turn *autocatalyzes* the activation of other pepsinogen molecules (Fig. 6.4a). When the pH exceeds 5, then pepsin becomes denatured. Hence, pepsin becomes denatured in the duodenum with the addition of bicarbonate in the pancreatic fluids (Fig. 6.4b). The pancreatic acinar cells (see Fig. 4.6) are the source for a variety of protein digestive enzymes including *trypsin, chymotrypsin, carboxypeptidase A and B*, and *elastase*. Cholecystokinin triggers the secretion of these pancreatic proteases, in inactive forms, that are activated in the small intestine (Fig. 6.4b). The brush border enzyme, *enteropeptidase*, activates trypsinogen to trypsin, which then activates chymotrypsinogen to chymotrypsin, procarboxypeptidase A & B to carboxypeptidase A & B, and proelastase to elastase. Trypsin also activates more molecules of trypsinogen to trypsin to accelerate the digestive process. Upon completion of their digestive action, the peptidases digest themselves as well. The digestive products include free amino acids, dipeptides, tripeptides, and oligopeptides (up to eight amino acids). The intestinal mucosa provides the other major source of protein digestive enzymes, namely, amino-oligopeptidase, dipeptidase, and enteropeptidase. It is important to note that the intestinal mucosa peptidases are mostly brush border, membrane bound and that the peptide transporters are Na^+ dependent as described below.

Reality check 6-2: Gastric cancer patients who undergo total gastric resection are still able to digest and absorb proteins. Why?

Reality check 6-3: Patients with Zollinger–Ellison syndrome (gastric acid hypersecretory state) may present with disturbances in protein absorption. Why?

6.3.5   Recall Points

Digestion of Proteins
- Chief cells of the stomach secrete pepsinogen (inactive precursor).
- Gastric pH converts pepsinogen into pepsin via autoactivation.
- Pepsin autocatalyzes the activation of more pepsinogen to pepsin.
- Pepsin is not essential for protein digestion.
- Pancreatic proteases are secreted in inactive forms.
- Enteropeptidase, a brush border enzyme, activates trypsinogen to trypsin.
- Trypsin activates the pancreatic protease precursors to their active forms.
- Hydrolysis of proteins produces amino acids, and di-, tri-, and oligo-peptides.

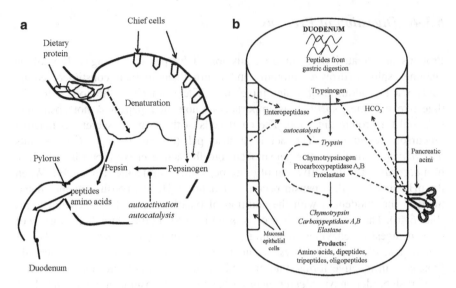

Fig. 6.4 Digestion of dietary protein. (**a**) Dietary protein is denatured by gastric acid making it available for potential hydrolysis by pepsin, the activated form of pepsinogen. Pepsinogen, which is secreted by gastric chief cells, autoactivates in the presence of stomach acid to pepsin, which in turn autocatalyzes the activation of more pepsinogen molecules. Large peptide fragments and small amounts of amino acids then move to the duodenum. (**b**) Peptides are hydrolyzed by a variety of proteases secreted in their inactive zymogen forms by pancreatic acinar cells. Enteropeptidase from mucosal epithelial cells activates trypsinogen to trypsin, which then activates chymotrypsinogen, pro-carboxypeptidases, and proelastase, as well as more trypsinogen, to their active forms. Free amino acids and di-, tri-, and oligopeptides are produced for final processing. Bicarbonate is also secreted from the pancreas to neutralize stomach acid

6.3.6   Digestion of Lipids

Neutral fats (also known as triglycerides) are the most abundant source of dietary fats. Neutral fats are provided primarily by animal sources compared to plant sources. There are several sources of digestive enzymes for lipids including preduodenal lipases (food-bearing lipases), lingual lipase, gastric lipase, and pancreatic lipase. Food-bearing lipases (e.g., phospholipases) and acid lipases may function in the autodigestion of food, a process which is facilitated by the acid environment of the stomach. For example, maternal milk contains a lipase that is identical to bile salt-stimulated lipase secreted by the pancreas. The saliva provides lingual lipase, which is secreted in the mouth by the lingual glands and swallowed with the saliva. In the stomach, a small amount of triglycerides can be digested by lingual lipase. The presence of chyme in the duodenum stimulates the secretion of CCK from I cells and results in the slowing of gastric emptying.

The pancreas is the source for *lipase, colipase, phospholipase A₂*, and *cholesterol ester hydrolase*. The majority of lipid digestion takes place in the small intestine via the action of pancreatic lipases. Pancreatic lipase (glycerol-ester lipase) is optimally active at pH 8 and maintains activity down to pH 3. Secreted in an active form, pancreatic lipase is destroyed in a more acidic environment and its enzymatic activity is inhibited by bile salts. However, the inhibition of pancreatic lipase activity is prevented under physiological conditions by the interaction of colipase with lipase. Colipase is secreted as a procolipase by the pancreas along with lipase in a 1:1 ratio. Procolipase is activated following its hydrolysis by trypsin. As noted above trypsinogen, secreted by the pancreas along with pancreatic lipases, is activated to trypsin by enteropeptidase. The presence of fat, mediated by cholecystokinin, stimulates the secretion of lipase–colipase complexes in the duodenum in large quantities. Bile salts inactivate lipase by displacing lipase at the fat droplet–water interface where lipase exerts its action. Colipase prevents the inactivation of lipase by bile salts by taking the place of bile salts at the fat droplet–water interface, thus allowing for the breakdown of triglycerides.

Emulsification is a key process in fat digestion. Initially, fat is broken down into smaller sized globules by agitation in the stomach and the addition in the duodenum of hepatic bile which contains bile salts and lecithin, and results in the breakdown of fat into even smaller sized globules (Fig. 6.5). Emulsification results in the dispersal of small fat droplets in the aqueous solution of the intestine and results in an increased surface area for the action of the pancreatic digestive enzymes.

Triglycerides via the action of food bearing, lingual, gastric, and pancreatic lipases are broken down into 2-monoglycerides and fatty acids. Cholesterol esters in the presence of cholesterol ester hydrolase are broken down into cholesterol and fatty acids. Phospholipids are digested by phospholipase A_2 to yield lysolecithin and fatty acid.

Reality check 6-4: You are asked to see Mr. Stephenson, a 49-year-old man with chronic pancreatitis secondary to alcohol abuse. While eliciting his GI review of symptoms, you note that he complains of greasy, diarrheal bowel movements. Why?

6.3.7 Recall Points

Digestion of Lipids
- Triglycerides are neutral fats and the most abundant dietary source of fats.
- Neutral fats are provided primarily by animal sources.
- Majority of lipid digestion takes place in the small intestine via the action of pancreatic lipases.
- Emulsification results in an increased surface area for the action of the pancreatic digestive enzymes.

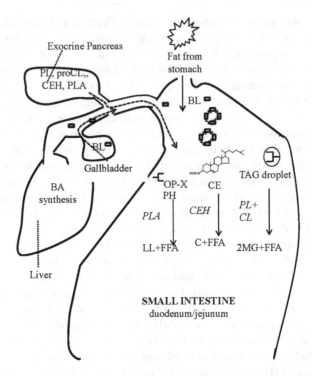

Fig. 6.5 Emulsification of dietary fat. Fat from the stomach is emulsified with bile salts and lecithin (BL; *small rectangles*) in the duodenum. Bile salts are converted from bile acids (BA) synthesized in the liver. The emulsified fat is digested by several lipases secreted from the pancreas. Pancreatic lipase (*PL*) hydrolyzes triacylglycerols (TAG) to 2-monoacylglycerol (2MG) plus free fatty acids (FFA) in the presence of colipase (*CL*). CL is also secreted from the pancreas but in an inactive procolipase (proCL) form that is activated by the action of trypsin (not shown). Cholesterol ester (CE) is de-esterified by cholesterol ester hydrolase (*CEH*) to cholesterol plus FFA. Phospholipids (PH) are hydrolyzed by phospholipase A2 (*PLA*) to lysolecithin (LL) and FFA. Like CL, PLA is activated from its inactive "pro" form (pPLA) by trypsin

6.4   Absorption

The process of gastrointestinal absorption occurs by active transport, diffusion, and in some cases *solvent drag* in which the flow of solvent drags dissolved substances along. Most gastrointestinal tract absorption occurs in the small intestine and entails between 7 and 8 L of water, several hundred grams of carbohydrates, 100 or more grams of fat, and 50–100 grams of both amino acids and ions. It is important to note that the small intestine has the capacity to absorb a greater amount than the above-noted substances. The large intestine absorbs only a few nutrients, but it can absorb additional amounts of water and ions.

6.4.1 Absorption of Carbohydrates

Glucose and galactose are absorbed from the intestinal lumen into the epithelial cells via a Na^+-dependent cotransport process (Fig. 6.6). Using the *sodium–glucose transport system* (SGLT), the glucose and galactose are actively transported against their concentration gradient or "uphill," while the sodium is transported along its concentration or "downhill." The Na^+–K^+ pump located in the basolateral cell membrane keeps the intracellular sodium level low and maintains the sodium gradient across the luminal membrane. Fructose transport into the epithelial cells occurs via the GLUT-5 transporter solely by facilitated diffusion. Hence, fructose cannot be transported against a concentration gradient. Glucose can also be absorbed via GLUT-5 though the SGLT mechanism is preferred. Glucose, galactose, and fructose exit across the basolateral membrane of the cell into the blood via facilitated diffusion using the GLUT-2 transporter.

Malabsorption of carbohydrates generally occurs when ingested carbohydrates are not broken down into the absorbable monosaccharides form. Patients who have lactose intolerance lack the brush border lactase enzyme that degrades this milk sugar. Hence, the nonabsorbable lactose disaccharide attracts water into the gut lumen and the patient experiences an osmotic diarrhea. Similarly certain populations (e.g., Inuits) exhibit trehalose intolerance and hence cannot properly digest fungi (e.g., mushrooms).

Reality check 6-5: You are studying the gastrointestinal absorption of carbohydrates (glucose and galactose) in a rat model. During the course of your experiments you apply a potent inhibitor of the Na^+–K^+ pump. Subsequently, you notice that it takes the rat a longer period of time to traverse a frequently traveled maze. You deduce that the rat is suffering from some form of cognitive impairment (a known side effect of hypoglycemia). Why?

Reality check 6-6: You are taking call for the local college student infirmary. A student presents with gaseousness and bloating due to lactose intolerance. Briefly describe two possible mechanisms for lactose intolerance.

6.4.2 Recall Points

Absorption of Carbohydrates
- Carbohydrates must be in the form of monosaccharides in order to be absorbed in the GI tract.
- Glucose and galactose enter the intestinal epithelial cell by Na^+-dependent cotransport and exit the cell by facilitated diffusion.
- Fructose enters the intestinal cell by facilitated diffusion and exits the cell by facilitated diffusion.
- Monosaccharides cross the basolateral membrane by facilitated diffusion.

Fig. 6.6 Intestinal absorption of monosaccharides. Monosaccharides are derived from the hydrolysis of dietary amylose, amylopectin, and disaccharides, as well as fructose. Glucose and galactose are absorbed by cotransport with Na^+ via sodium–glucose transporter (SGLT). The Na^+–K^+-ATPase pump (ATP) maintains a low intracellular Na^+ concentration. Fructose and glucose are absorbed passively via the GLUT-5 (G5) transporter. All the monosaccharides diffuse passively into the blood via the GLUT-2 transporter (G2)

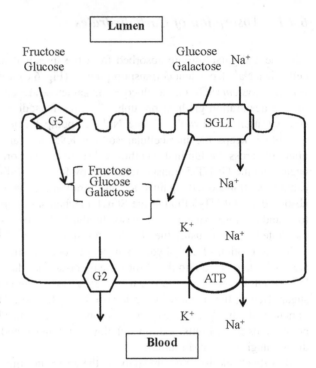

6.4.3 Absorption of Amino Acids

Proteases digest dietary proteins into more absorbable dipeptides, tripeptides, and amino acids. Dipeptides and tripeptides are the most frequently absorbed protein digestion products as compared to free amino acids. The intestinal brush border membrane contains a single peptide transport system that mediates the absorption of di- and tripeptides (Fig. 6.7). The approximately 20 different amino acids that constitute dietary proteins are not transported individually by this di- and tripeptide-specific transport system. The combined action of the Na^+–H^+ exchanger in the brush border membrane together with the Na^+–K^+-ATPase in the enterocyte basolateral membrane generates and maintains a H^+ electrochemical gradient across the brush border membrane and a microclimate acid pH region on the luminal surface of the intestinal brush border membrane (see Fig. 4.9a). The generation of an electrochemical H^+ gradient is used to transport di- and tripeptides rather than a transmembrane electrochemical Na^+ gradient. This peptide transport system transports di- and tripeptides consisting of anionic amino acids, cationic amino acids, and neutral amino acids. Once inside the cell, cytosolic di- and tripeptidases hydrolyze the majority of the dipeptides and tripeptides to produce amino acids that exit the cell across the basolateral membrane via facilitated diffusion (Fig. 6.7). To accommodate the variety of amino acid side chain characteristics, the intestinal brush border membrane contains at least seven distinct

Fig. 6.7 Intestinal absorption of amino acids. Most amino acids are absorbed as dipeptides or tripeptides that are hydrolyzed by peptidases in the epithelial cells. Their uptake depends on a H^+ gradient created by the Na^+–H^+ exchanger. Individual amino acids are absorbed via Na^+-dependent cotransport driven by the Na^+–K^+-ATPase pump (ATP) that maintains a low intracellular Na^+ concentration

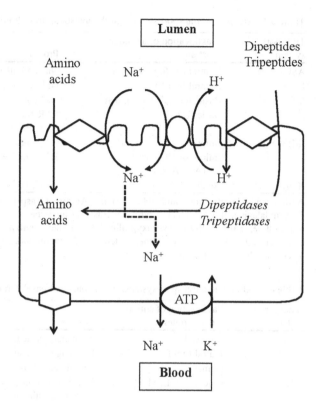

amino acid transport systems for which there is overlap of specificity (Table 6.1). Most of these amino acid transport systems involve Na^+-dependent carriers tied to the Na^+–K^+-ATPase pump (Fig. 6.7), while others use exchange with neutral amino acids or a H^+-cotransport system (PAT) like the peptide transporter. In general, though, there is a significant difference between the peptide and amino acid absorptive processes in terms of their source of energy; H^+ and Na^+ electrochemical gradients, respectively.

Once free amino acids are present in the intestinal cell cytoplasm either through amino acid transport or through the action of cytosolic peptidases on di- and tripeptides, the free amino acids may enter various metabolic pathways, e.g., degradation, incorporation into other proteins, conversion to other amino acids, and/or incorporation into cellular proteins. Free amino acids in the cytoplasm of the enterocyte enter the portal circulation via four specific basolateral membrane amino acid transport systems that differ from those in the brush border membrane (Table 6.2). During periods of feeding, the basolateral membrane amino acid transport systems export amino acids from the enterocyte into the portal circulation. In contrast, during periods when amino acids are not available from the intestinal lumen (e.g., between meals), the intestinal basolateral membrane amino acid transport systems import amino acids from the portal circulation into the enterocyte for cellular metabolism.

Table 6.1 Amino acid transport systems in the intestinal brush border (apical) membrane

Transport system	Classification of amino acid substrates	Process
ASC	Neutral (A, S, C, T, Q only)	Na^+-cotransport
B^0	Neutral (not P)	Na^+-cotransport
B^{0+}	Basic, neutral (not P), β-A	Na^+-cotransport
b^{0+}	Basic (H?)	K, R Na^+-cotransport; others exchange with neutral amino acids
IMINO	Imino	Na^+-cotransport
PAT	Imino, small neutral (A, β-A, G)	H^+-cotransport
X^-_{AG}	Acidic	$2Na^+$, $1H^+$-cotransport and $1K^+$ exchange

Amino acid classifications and abbreviations: **Acidic:** *D* aspartate, *E* glutamate; **Aromatic:** *F* phenylalanine, *W* tryptophan, *Y* tyrosine; **Basic:** *H* histidine, *K* lysine, *O* ornithine, *R* arginine, *S-S* cystine; **Imino:** *HO-P* hydroxyproline, *P* proline; **Neutral:** *A* alanine, *β-A* β-alanine, *C* cysteine, *G* glycine, *I* isoleucine, *L* leucine, *M* methionine, *N* asparagine, *Q* glutamine, *S* serine, *T* threonine, *V* valine

Table 6.2 Amino acid transport systems in the intestinal basolateral membrane

Transport system	Classification of amino acid substrates	Process
ASC	A, C, S, T	Exchange for neutral extracellular amino acid
L	Neutral (not P)	Exchange for neutral extracellular amino acid
T	Aromatic	Facilitated diffusion
y^+L	Basic; A, C, L, M, Q	K, R Na^+-cotransport; others exchange for neutral extracellular amino acid

Amino acid classifications and abbreviations—see Table 6.1

Clinical Implications: Drug Interactions. There are a variety of possible clinical implications of peptide and free amino acid assimilation. Absorption of protein digestion products occurs predominantly in the form of small peptides rather than free amino acids. The intestinal peptide transporter may interact with several pharmacologically significant drugs which have peptide-like chemical structures. These drugs undergo efficient absorption when taken orally due to the peptide transporter. Hence, the peptide transporter system may have a significant effect upon the bioavailability of peptidomimetic drugs. The efficacy of peptide-based formula solutions is facilitated by the intestinal peptide absorption process because amino acids are absorbed more efficiently from peptides than from an equivalent mixture of free amino acids.

Clinical Implications: Pancreatic Disease. Inadequacy in the amount or function of pancreatic enzymes or intestinal epithelial cell transporters results in abnormalities in protein digestion and absorption. Patients with chronic pancreatitis and exocrine pancreatic insufficiency do not produce enough digestive enzymes, e.g., peptidases. Hence, ingested proteins cannot be broken down into absorbable dipeptides, tripeptides, and amino acids.

Clinical Implications: Inherited Transport System Disorders. Patients with *cystinuria* have a defect in the b^{0+} transporter system for the dibasic amino acids arginine, cystine, lysine, and ornithine. These patients are unable to absorb the dibasic amino acids due to an intestinal defect and hence excrete them in the stool. The identical transporter is found in renal epithelial cells resulting in the increased excretion of the specific dibasic amino acid. Because of its lower solubility, in particular cystine is excreted in the urine (cystinuria) and may precipitate in the kidney forming cystine stones. *Hartnup* disorder is characterized by a defect of the B^0 transport system for neutral amino acids.

Reality check 6-7: A patient presents with protein malabsorption. How might you clinically distinguish whether the patient's problem is due to an insufficient amount or activity level of pancreatic proteases versus a problem with insufficient activity or levels of transporters for intestinal epithelial cell transporters?

Case in Point 6-1

Chief Complaint: A 2-month-old male is admitted to the hospital for dehydration associated with persistent diarrhea.

History: The patient was a full-term infant with a birth weight of 3.6 kg. There were no complications reported with labor or delivery. Family history is unremarkable. The patient is not taking any medications and has not had any sick contacts. The patient has no history of fever, vomiting, or hematochezia (blood in feces). Attempts to breast-feed the patient early in life were unsuccessful secondary to diarrhea that began on day 4 of life. When oral intake was stopped, there was quick resolution of the diarrhea. The patient had been tried on multiple formulas including cow's milk-based, partial hydrolysate (treated with *Lactobacillus acidophilus*) but the symptoms were not relieved by this diet.

Physical Exam: On examination, the patient is in the 10th percentile for weight and length. He shows no acute distress. His mucous membranes are mildly dry and he is anicteric (not jaundiced). Lungs and heart exam are normal. The abdomen is soft, nondistended, and without hepatosplenomegaly. Neurological, musculoskeletal, and skin exams are normal. The stool is negative for occult blood.

Labs:

Hb 16.3 g/dL [*N*: 14.7–18.6]	Hct 49 % [*N*: 43–56 %]
RBC 5.1×10^6 cells/µL [*N*: 4.2–5.5]	WBC 10.1×10^3 cells/µL [*N*: 6.8–13.3]
Platelets 250×10^9 cells/L [*N*: 164–351]	Albumin 2.4 g/dL [*N*: 2.6–3.6]
Sodium 140 mEq/L [*N*: 133–146]	Potassium 4.0 mEq/L [*N*: 3.7–5.2]
Chloride 101 mEq/L [*N*: 96–111]	Bicarbonate 21 mM [*N*: 19–24]

Stool Analysis: routine culture, ova and parasite testing, *Clostridium difficile* toxin are negative, positive for reducing substances with a pH of 5.

(continued)

Imaging: upper endoscopy and flexible sigmoidoscopy revealed no histo-
logic abnormalities.
Other: Hydrogen breath testing after ingesting galactose as the substrate.
Control = hydrogen at 5 ppm.

Time = 45 min	Hydrogen = 45 ppm
Time = 90 min	Hydrogen = 20 ppm
Time = 120 min	Hydrogen = 5 ppm

Assessment: On the basis of the findings does this patient have a secretory
diarrhea or an osmotic diarrhea and what is the basis for your conclusion?
What is the significance of the stool being positive for reducing substances? What is the significance of the finding that giving the infant
cow's milk-based partial hydrolysate (treated with *Lactobacillus acidophilus*) formula did not relieve the symptoms? What is your diagnosis?

6.4.4   Recall Points

Absorption of Proteins
• Dipeptides and tripeptides are the most frequently absorbed protein digestion
  products.
• Dipeptides and tripeptides enter the intestinal epithelial cell via H^+-dependent
  cotransport that uses a H^+ electrochemical gradient.
• Cytosolic peptidases hydrolyze dipeptides and tripeptides into amino acids.
• Seven different amino acid transport systems with overlapping specificity oper-
  ate in the apical membrane mostly via a Na^+-cotransport mechanism that uses a
  Na^+ electrochemical gradient.
• Amino acids leave the cell via four different amino acid transport systems that
  utilize facilitated diffusion or exchange transport.

6.4.5   Absorption of Lipids

The absorption of lipids takes place in several steps. First, the breakdown products of
lipid digestion, monoglycerides, free fatty acids, lysolecithin, and cholesterol are
mixed with the amphipathic bile salts to form mixed micelles (see Fig. 4.7). The
center of the micelle contains the lipid digestion products, while the hydrophilic
portions of the micelles dissolve in the aqueous component of the intestinal lumen
(see Fig. 5.3). Second, the micelles travel to the apical brush border of the intestinal

epithelial cells and release the lipid digestion products (see Fig. 4.8). The micelles do not enter the cells and the bile salts are absorbed further down the GI tract in the ileum. Third, once inside the intestinal epithelial cells, the lipid products of digestion are reesterified with free fatty acids to form phospholipids, cholesterol ester, and triglycerides. Fourth, the reesterified lipids combined with apoproteins to form chylomicrons. Fifth, the chylomicrons migrate to the basolateral membrane of the epithelial cell of the small intestine, and exocytosis of the chylomicrons occurs. Because the chylomicrons are too large to enter into the capillaries they enter into the lacteals and subsequently the thoracic duct and ultimately the blood (see Fig. 4.8).

There are several possible scenarios that could interfere with lipid absorption: (1) In the presence of an increased acid load in the duodenum, the neutralizing ability of bicarbonate is overcome, and pancreatic lipase is rendered inactive. (2) In patients who suffer from pancreatic insufficiency, the amount of bicarbonate secreted by the pancreas may be insufficient to neutralize the H^+ present. Hence, the pancreatic lipases will fail to function appropriately. (3) Interruption of the enterohepatic circulation or a deficiency of bile salts results in a reduced amount of micelles, which in turn can lead to an impairment of lipid absorption. Alternately a reduction of the intestinal lumen pH can contribute to the early absorption of bile acids because they will exist in their nonionized form. The reduction of the number of micelles due to the early absorption of bile acids would impair lipid absorption. Additionally, bacterial overgrowth results in the deconjugation of bile salts converting them into their nonionized bile acid forms and attendant early absorption of bile acids. (4) Chylomicrons are critical to the transport of lipids out of the intestinal cells into the thoracic duct and blood. Patients with *abetalipoproteinemia* do not produce Apo B48 and hence assembly and thus transport of lipids normally contained in chylomicrons becomes impaired. (5) When a patient suffers a reduction of intestinal cells for absorption whether due to surgical resection, ablation, or infiltration of the intestinal wall by a connective tissue disorder, tumor, infection, or inflammation, then lipid absorption will be compromised.

Reality check 6-8: You have just completed a history and physical exam on a patient with celiac disease (an autoimmune disorder of the small bowel due to a reaction to a gluten protein named gliadin). During your elicitation of the patient's review of symptoms, you note that he complains of fatigue, weight loss, and diarrhea. When you look up celiac disease on your PDA, you note that the small bowel biopsy of these patients shows blunting of villi, crypt hyperplasia, and lymphocyte infiltration of crypts. Briefly describe two possible causes for lipid malabsorption in celiac disease.

6.4.6 Recall Points

Absorption of Lipids
- Products of lipid digestion mix with bile salts to form mixed micelles.
- Micelles release the lipid breakdown products at the apical brush border of the intestinal epithelial cells.

- Inside the epithelial cells, the lipid breakdown products are reesterified with free fatty acids to form lipids again.
- Reesterified lipids combine with apoproteins to form chylomicrons.
- Chylomicrons undergo exocytosis and enter into the lacteals, and subsequently the thoracic duct and blood.

6.4.7 Absorption of Calcium, Iron, and Vitamins

Vitamin D is activated in the kidney from the 25-OH-cholecalciferol form by parathyroid hormone to its 1,25-$(OH)_2$cholecalciferol form. The activated vitamin D enhances the absorption of calcium from the small intestine (see Fig. 4.11). In the small intestine, it causes the formation of calbindin D-28K intestinal Ca^{2+}-binding protein. Patients with chronic renal failure or vitamin D deficiency produce insufficient amounts of calbindin D-28K intestinal Ca^{2+}-binding protein and hence cannot absorb sufficient amounts of calcium. In children this deficiency leads to rickets while in adults insufficient vitamin D causes osteomalacia.

The absorption of iron plays a critical role in the maintenance of a stable level of 4 grams in healthy adults. Total body iron requirements and the bioavailability of iron regulate the process. Sloughing of GI tract and skin cells leads to the loss of 1–2 mg/day of iron. In general, because body iron is conserved, the amount of iron absorbed by the intestine is less than the amount ingested. The recommended daily intake of iron is 20 mg/day. However, women absorb only 1.0–1.5 mg/day and men absorb only 0.5–1.0 mg/day. The main sources of dietary iron are heme (derived from meat) and inorganic iron (predominantly Fe^{2+}). Intestinal cells absorb heme via endocytosis (see Fig. 4.12). Next, cytosolic enzymes release Fe^{2+} from the heme molecule.

The absorption of nonheme iron (the largest fraction of dietary iron) occurs by a different mechanism. In the presence of gastric acid, the insoluble complexes of iron with food become more soluble. Namely, iron is released from food in the more soluble Fe^{2+} form as opposed to the less soluble Fe^{3+} form. Free dietary iron that is in the ferric (oxidized) state must first be reduced in the intestinal lumen by *ferric reductase* to the ferrous form (Fe^{2+}) prior to absorption. Enterocytes of the proximal small intestine secrete transferrin (iron binding protein) which binds two iron ions in the lumen. The iron–transferrin complex binds to the enterocytes brush border membrane receptor and is absorbed via the *divalent metal transporter* in the apical membrane (see Fig. 4.12).

Once inside the enterocyte, some of the iron derived from heme or nonheme sources is bound to ferritin and stored in the cell. Most of the remaining freed iron is bound to transferrin and enters the blood by an unknown process.

Iron absorption is adjusted and regulated by the body's needs. For example, *hemochromatosis* represents an iron overload disorder that can occur due to excess iron absorption. To prevent excess iron absorption, ferritin (iron storage protein) is upregulated in the enterocyte cytoplasm leading to an increased formation of iron/

Table 6.3 The B vitamins

Vitamin	Common name	Cofactor forms
1	Thiamine	Thiamine pyrophosphate
2	Riboflavin	Flavin adenine dinucleotide (FAD) or flavin mononucleotide (FMN)
3	Niacin	Nicotinamide adenine dinucleotide (NAD) or nicotinamide adenine dinucleotide phosphate (NADP)
5	Pantothenic acid	Coenzyme A
6	Pyridoxine	Pyridoxal phosphate
7	Biotin	Biotin covalently attached to a lysine residue
9	Folic acid	Tetrahydrofolate modified with single carbon units
12	Cobalamin	Methylcobalamin and adenosylcobalamin

ferritin complexes, which are lost in the feces when the intestinal epithelial cells are sloughed off. Additionally, the rate of iron absorption can be decreased by the reduction of the number of receptors for the transferrin/iron complexes on the brush borders of the enterocytes. On the other hand, as a consequence of blood loss (e.g., during menses) or pregnancy, additional iron is required by the body. Hence, the amount of ferritin is downregulated, and the enterocyte brush border receptors for the transferrin/iron complexes are increased in numbers.

The B vitamins (Table 6.3) are all water soluble vitamins. In general, absorption of water soluble vitamins occurs by a Na^+-dependent cotransport process in the small bowel. However, vitamin B12 requires intrinsic factor as described in Chap. 4 (see Fig. 4.3).

Connecting-the-Dots 6-1

A 23-year-old man with cystic fibrosis (CF) comes to the Internal Medicine Clinic complaining of cough, abdominal pain, and steatorrhea. CF is a hereditary disorder in which most exocrine glands produce abnormal mucus that obstructs glands and ducts. On physical examination, he appears fatigued and in mild respiratory distress. The respiratory rate is 26/min, and his breath sounds are decreased. The abdominal exam is notable for mild-to-moderate tenderness to deep palpation in the midepigastric region. Laboratory findings reveal moderate-to-severe pancreatic dysfunction characterized by low serum levels of amylase, lipase, total proteins, and increased fecal fat. In addition, chest radiogram shows bronchiectasis, and airflow obstruction is noted on spirometry. As you read further in the patient's chart you see that the patient has had a complete pulmonary and GI work-up and was diagnosed with stable COPD and pancreatic insufficiency. A pert second-year nursing student who is assisting you asks you what you want to do about the patient's malabsorption symptoms.

6.5 Summary Points

- Digestion occurs when food is broken up through the action of the teeth or through the chemical action of enzymes and converted into a substance suitable for absorption or excretion.
- Human digestion occurs primarily in the small intestine.
- Hydrolysis is the main chemical process involved in the digestion of all major nutrients.
- Absorption is the uptake of substances by a tissue across the wall of the intestine.
- Carbohydrates must be broken down to the monosaccharides (glucose, galactose, and fructose) in order for absorption to take place.
- Glucose and galactose are absorbed from the intestinal lumen into the cells by a Na^+-dependent cotransport process and they are transported from inside the cell to the blood by facilitated diffusion.
- Fructose transport is solely mediated by facilitated diffusion.
- Pepsin is produced in the stomach and is not essential for protein digestion due to the roles played by pancreatic proteases and the intestinal mucosa which is a major source of amino-oligopeptidase, dipeptidase, and enteropeptidase.
- Pancreatic proteases are secreted in inactive forms.
- Enteropeptidase (brush border enzyme) activates trypsinogen to trypsin, which sets off activation cascade of inactive pancreatic proteases.
- Triglycerides are neutral fats and the most abundant source of dietary fats.
- Chyme in the duodenum stimulates production of CCK from I cells and slows gastric emptying.
- Majority of lipid digestion occurs in the small bowel due to the action of pancreatic lipases.
- Emulsification of fats increases the surface area for the action of pancreatic digestive enzymes.
- The monosaccharides glucose and galactose are actively absorbed by a Na^+-dependent cotransport at the luminal membrane and exit the cell by facilitated diffusion.
- Lactose intolerance is due to either insufficient or inactive lactase brush border enzyme.
- Di- and tripeptides are the most frequently absorbed products of protein digestion which enter the intestinal cells by H^+-dependent cotransport mechanism.
- Cytosolic peptidases hydrolyze most di- and tripeptides to produce amino acids which leave the cell by facilitated diffusion.
- Patients with pancreatic insufficiency do not produce peptidases in sufficient numbers or with sufficient levels of activity which results in protein malabsorption.
- Micelles travel to the brush border of the intestinal epithelial cell and release the lipids. Micelles do not enter the cells.

- Reesterified lipids combine with apoproteins to form chylomicrons which migrate to the basolateral membrane of the intestinal cell and undergo exocytosis in order to enter into the lacteals and ultimately the blood.
- Bile salts are absorbed in the ileum.
- Bacterial overgrowth leads to the deconjugation of bile salts which results in bile acid conversion to their nonionized form and attendant early absorption.
- Chronic renal failure or vitamin D-deficient patients cannot produce sufficient amounts of calbindin D-28K intestinal Ca^{2+}-binding protein and therefore cannot absorb sufficient amounts of calcium, thus producing rickets in children and osteomalacia in adults.
- Water soluble vitamins (B1, B2, B6, pantothenic acid, nicotinic acid, folic acid, and biotin) undergo absorption via a Na^+-dependent cotransport process in the small bowel. Vitamin B12 requires intrinsic factor for absorption.

6.6 Review Questions

6-1. An 18-year-old coed presents to the college infirmary with an acute viral syndrome. During your elicitation of her GI review of symptoms, she complains of a new onset of lactose intolerance. Which of the following recommendations would you include for this patient?

A. No recommendation to avoid intake of any foods
B. Permanent avoidance of dairy products
C. Permanent avoidance of fruit
D. Permanent avoidance of mushrooms
E. Temporary avoidance of dairy products
F. Temporary avoidance of fruit
G. Temporary avoidance of mushrooms

6-2. A 25-year-old medical student complains of gaseousness, bloating, and diarrhea every time she consumes milk products. Which of the following most likely accurately describes the primary cause of this patient's intolerance to milk products?

A. Decreased activity of the glucoamylase brush border enzyme
B. Decreased activity of the lactase brush border enzyme
C. Decreased activity of the sucrose–isomaltase brush border enzyme complex
D. Defect in the Na^+-dependent galactose transporter
E. Defect in the Na^+-dependent glucose transporter

6-3. Ms. Jolie is a 32-year-old woman who is referred for diarrhea after gallbladder surgery. Her past medical history is significant for an uncomplicated pregnancy and hyperlipidemia. After a thorough gastrointestinal evaluation you diagnose bile salt-induced diarrhea and start her on cholestyramine, a bile salt binding agent. Which of the following situations will this patient most likely experience?

A. Decrease in her serum lipids
B. Increase in her bile salt pool
C. Increase in her serum lipids
D. No changes in her bile salt pool

6-4. You are asked to see an infant in the pediatric clinic with Bassen–Kornzweig syndrome (abetalipoproteinemia). The infant has a history of diarrhea and foul smelling stools. Physical exam reveals failure to thrive and abdominal bloating. Which of the following conditions will most likely be true for this patient?

A. Patient's blood level of fat soluble vitamins will be elevated
B. Patient's blood level of water soluble vitamins will be elevated
C. Patient's stool will contain a decreased amount of fat
D. Patient's stool will contain an increased amount of fat

6-5. Which of the following statements regarding intestinal vitamin absorption is correct?

A. All the B vitamins require intrinsic factor for absorption
B. Fat soluble vitamin absorption occurs by a Na^+-dependent cotransport process in the small bowel
C. Iron absorption in the small intestine occurs primarily in the terminal ileum
D. Patients with chronic renal failure or vitamin D deficiency generally cannot absorb sufficient amounts of calcium

6.7   Answer to Case in Point

Case in Point 6-1: An important aspect of this patient's presentation is the resolution of symptoms when restricted from any oral intake. When considering the work-up for diarrhea it is important to distinguish between an osmotic diarrhea and a secretory diarrhea because the differential diagnosis between the two is drastically different. With an osmotic diarrhea, the intestinal mucosa is often damaged and cannot digest and absorb nutrients. In a special case of osmotic diarrhea, carbohydrate malabsorption, there may be no direct damage to intestinal mucosa but rather the absence of necessary transporters for the absorption of monosaccharides or the congenital absence of enzymes needed to break down complex carbohydrates. Because of this, an osmotic gradient is established that drives water into the lumen, leading to diarrhea. In contrast, a secretory diarrhea occurs because the intestinal epithelial cells are turned into a state of active secretion leading to active transport of ions and water into the lumen of the intestine. The differential diagnosis for secretory diarrhea includes several infectious agents, including toxin-producing bacteria (cholera); neuroendocrine secreting tumors; and a congenital defect in the transport of chloride, congenital chloridorrhea. Based on the patient's history of resolution of symptoms when enteric feedings were removed, an osmotic diarrhea was suspected.

When considering chronic diarrhea of infancy secondary to an osmotic process, one should consider several diagnoses. An infectious agent, either viral or bacterial, can cause damage to the intestinal mucosal lining and produce a protracted diarrheal illness. Milk protein allergy, which often presents from a few days to a few weeks after the introduction of milk protein into the diet, can cause symptoms ranging from irritability and hematochezia to diarrhea and vomiting. Casein hydrolysate formulas are usually therapeutic, although severely affected infants may require an amino acid-based formula. Breast-fed infants, despite no direct exposure to cow's milk protein, can still develop an allergy as the milk protein is expressed in breast milk. Other less common causes, including carbohydrate intolerance from congenital enzymatic abnormalities or transporter defects, microvillus inclusion disease, and autoimmune enteropathy, should also be considered.

Additional testing, including stool and serum osmolality as well as stool electrolytes, would be performed if the diagnosis is in question. As noted, the patient had an osmotic diarrhea with a negative work-up for infectious agents, endoscopy that showed no evidence of inflammation or other abnormalities, and stool that was positive for reducing substances with an acidic pH. Of the diagnoses that remain, carbohydrate intolerance is the most likely. With this group of disorders, endoscopy is macroscopically and microscopically normal. Instead, one needs to consider the use of disaccharidase testing at the time of endoscopy, or hydrogen breath testing after ingestion of the suspected offending carbohydrate. That galactose produced elevated expiration of hydrogen suggested an inability to absorb galactose in the small intestine. Hence the diagnosis is a congenital galactose–glucose malabsorption syndrome caused by a defect of the SGLT-1 (sodium-dependent glucose transporter) in the intestine.

6.8   Answer to Connecting-the-Dots

Connecting-the-Dots 6-1: The abnormal mucus plugging of the pancreatic duct leads to chronic pancreatitis and subsequent pancreatic insufficiency. The pancreatic insufficiency results in a marked decrease in the production of amylase, lipase, and peptidases. This explains the patients abdominal pain (due to chronic pancreatitis), steatorrhea (increased fat in the stool due to lipid malabsorption), fatigue and weight loss (due to carbohydrate and protein malabsorption as well). The administration of pancreatic enzymes, especially lipase, will decrease fat malabsorption, as well as reverse the patient's weight loss and fatigue.

6.9 Answers to Reality Checks

Reality check 6-1: Sugar-free candies contain sugar alcohols, e.g., hexitols (sorbitol, mannitol, and xylitol), which are artificial sweeteners and are poorly absorbed from the intestinal lumen. These sugar alcohols are osmotically active and attract water into the lumen which results in diarrhea when consumed in excess.

Reality check 6-2: The stomach is the source for the digestive enzyme called pepsin. However, pepsin is not essential for protein digestion for the following reasons:

1. The pancreas is the source for trypsin, chymotrypsin, carboxypeptidase A & B, and elastase. These pancreatic digestive enzymes are secreted in inactive forms and are activated in the small intestine by the brush border enzyme, enterokinase which activates trypsinogen to trypsin. It should be noted that trypsin also activates trypsinogen to trypsin.
2. The intestinal mucosa provides the other major source of protein digestive enzymes, namely, amino-oligopeptidase, dipeptidase, and enterokinase.

Reality check 6-3: Excess gastric acid secretion causes inactivation of the pancreatic proteases and attendant protein malabsorption. In addition, hypersecretion of gastric acid causes diffuse ulceration of the intestine and results in a protein losing enteropathy.

Reality check 6-4: Excessive alcohol consumption is the most common cause of chronic pancreatitis in the USA and a very frequent cause of pancreatic insufficiency. Patients who suffer from chronic pancreatitis produce insufficient amounts of lipase which is crucial for the digestion of lipids. Malabsorption of lipids results in the excretion of greasy stools or steatorrhea.

Reality check 6-5: Glucose and galactose are absorbed from the intestinal lumen into the cells via a Na^+-dependent cotransport process. If one poisons the Na^+–K^+ pump, then nerve and muscle membrane function will be adversely affected. In addition, the absorption of glucose and galactose will be inhibited and the rat will experience hypoglycemia. Hence, the rat will have several causes of cognitive impairment which will result in it having a more difficult time negotiating the maze.

Reality check 6-6: A deficient amount or activity level of the lactase brush border enzyme will result in the malabsorption of lactose. In addition, if the patient had a deficient amount or insufficient activity level of the Na^+-dependent cotransporters then malabsorption of the breakdown products of lactose digestion (glucose and galactose) would also occur. It is important to note that in the case of insufficient levels or activity of the Na^+-dependent cotransporters, the patient would have problems with the absorption of lactose, glucose, and galactose.

Reality check 6-7: If the patient's protein malabsorption is due to insufficient amounts or low activity levels of pancreatic proteases, then if you either replace the pancreatic proteases or feed dipeptides and amino acids, the patient's protein malabsorption will correct. On the other hand, replacing pancreatic proteases will not help patients with a defect in intestinal epithelial cell transporters.

Reality check 6-8: Infiltration of the intestinal lining in the region of the terminal ileum as well as bowel wall edema (increased diffusion distance) will decrease the surface area for lipid absorption. Infiltration and edema of the bowel wall will impede the enterohepatic circulation of bile salts. Patients with diminished bile salts will absorb fewer lipids. In addition, you noted during your PDA search that celiac disease patients are prone to bacterial overgrowth. Bacterial overgrowth results in the deconjugation of bile salts which results in bile acids in their nonionized forms and attendant early absorption of bile acids.

6.10   Answers to Review Questions

6-1. **E.** The coed is suffering from an acute viral infection involving her gastrointestinal tract. The acute viral gastroenteritis will generally run its course in 4–5 days. At the end of 5 days, the coed's intestinal lining would have undergone reepithelialization and her brush border enzymes would be restored. Hence, by day 5 she should be able to digest lactose again. Temporary avoidance of dairy products during the initial days of her illness would help reduce the occurrence of lactose intolerant symptoms. Mushrooms contain trehalose, not lactose, and fruit contains the monosaccharide fructose.

6-2. **B.** Lactose intolerance is usually primarily due to a deficiency in either the amount or activity level of the lactase brush border enzyme. Lactose is digested into the monosaccharides glucose and galactose by lactase. If a patient had a defect in either the Na^+-dependent glucose or galactose transporters, then one would expect the patient to present with intolerance for various di- and monosaccharides as well as lactose. The sucrose–isomaltase complex acts on sucrose (table sugar), maltotriose, and α-limit dextrins (glucose oligosaccharide that includes a branch with an α-1,6 bond). The glucoamylase acts on oligosaccharides lacking an α-1,6 bond.

6-3. **A.** Cholestyramine is a bile salt binding agent which will reduce Ms. Jolie's bile salt pool. Hence, Ms. Jolie will have a reduced capacity to absorb lipids which will result in a lowering of her blood lipid levels.

6-4. **D.** Patients with abetalipoproteinemia have problems with lipid absorption. Hence, you would expect these patients to present with increased fat excretion in their stools. Their blood levels of fat soluble vitamins should be decreased whereas water soluble vitamins in the blood will be unaffected.

6-5. **D.** Patients with chronic renal failure or vitamin D deficiency cannot produce sufficient amounts of calbindin D-28K intestinal Ca^{2+}-binding protein. This in turn limits the absorption of calcium from the lumen of the small intestine. Only vitamin B12 requires intrinsic factor for absorption in the terminal ileum. Iron absorption occurs primarily in the duodenum. Water soluble vitamin absorption occurs via a Na^+-dependent cotransport process. Fat soluble vitamins diffuse into the intestinal enterocyte from mixed micelles. In the enterocyte they are incorporated into chylomicrons that enter the circulation from the thoracic duct via the lymphatics.

Suggested Reading

Janson LW, Tischler ME. The digestive system (Chapter 11). In: The big picture: medical biochemistry. New York: McGraw Hill; 2012. p. 149–66.

Kibble JD, Halsey CR. Gastrointestinal physiology (Chapter 7). In: The big picture: medical physiology. New York: McGraw Hill; 2009. p. 259–306.

Seifter J, Ratner A, Sloane D. Nutrition, digestion, and absorption (Chapter 27). In: Concepts in medical physiology. Philadelphia: Lippincott Williams & Williams; 2005. p. 425–52.

Chapter 7
Salt and Water: Intestinal Water and Electrolyte Transport

7.1 Introduction

There are important basic mechanisms involved in the absorption and secretion of water and electrolytes. Over a 24-h period, the intestinal tract secretes roughly 1.5 L of gastric secretions, 1 L each of saliva, pancreatic juice, and bile, 2 L of small intestinal secretion, and 0.2 L of large intestinal secretion; a sum of approximately 7 L of total secretions. Additionally, an average person consumes 1.5–2 L of dietary liquids per day. Thus, the gastrointestinal tract is presented with 9 L of fluid per day. All but 100–200 mL of the 9 L of intestinal fluids is absorbed in the small intestine and colon. The remaining intestinal fluids are excreted in the stools. Diarrhea results from incomplete absorption of intestinal fluids due to insufficient contact time with the intestinal absorptive epithelial surface or the lack of sufficient absorptive surface area. A full understanding of fluid and electrolyte transport requires an integrated study of the contributions made by the various regions of the gastrointestinal tract. The initial discussion of this complex topic focuses on the important role played by the proximal small intestine.

7.2 Functional Anatomy

The small intestine is approximately 22 ft in length allowing for significant contact time between the absorptive lining of the intestine, foodstuffs, and enzymes. *Plicae circulares* are the many folds of the mucosa and submucosa that are visible upon gross inspection of the bowel and that run transversely for two-thirds of the circumference of the gut (Fig. 7.1). The plicae circulares increase the absorptive surface area of the intestine approximately threefold. The jejunum has the greatest number of plicae circulares. Absorption of intestinal fluids occurs at the level of the epithelial lining cells of the villus and begins with the absorption of solute followed by fluid. Villi are finger-like projections of the mucosa and submucosa and increase

E. Trowers and M. Tischler, *Gastrointestinal Physiology*,
DOI 10.1007/978-3-319-07164-0_7, © Springer International Publishing Switzerland 2014

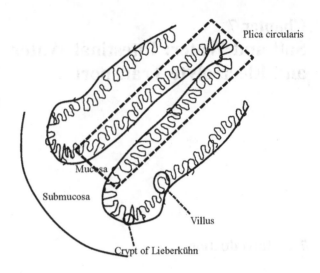

Fig. 7.1 Absorptive surface of the gut. The plicae circulares are the many folds of the intestinal mucosa and submucosa each of which contains numerous villi at the base of which are the Crypts of Lieberkühn

the absorptive surface area of the intestine tenfold. The base of the villi extends into the *Crypts of Lieberkühn*, which form tubular glands that open onto the intestinal lumen. Epithelial cells lining the crypts secrete electrolytes and fluids. In addition, the crypts contain stem cells that divide and give rise to epithelial and other intestinal cells. As the cells differentiate, they migrate from the crypts toward the tip of the villi surface. Migration continues until the cells are sloughed from the villi tips into the intestinal lumen. The exception to this migratory pattern is the lysozyme-producing paneth cells, which remain at the base of the crypts.

Microvilli are small finger-like projections located on the apical side of intestinal absorptive cells and increase the intestinal absorptive surface area approximately 20-fold (see Fig. 2.1). Digestive enzymes are bound to the microvilli membranes and hydrolyze complex peptides and carbohydrates into simple amino acids and sugars.

7.2.1   Recall Points

- Intestinal tract secretes 7 L of fluid in 24 h.
- The average person consumes 2 L of fluid daily.
- Plicae circulares, villi, and microvilli markedly increase the absorptive surface area of the intestinal tract.
- Material that enters the duodenum undergoes rapid osmotic equilibration with plasma.

Fig. 7.2 Absorption of water by intestinal cells. The hydrostatic pressure combined with the osmotic pressures in the intraepithelial space, interstitial space, and the capillaries favors the absorption of fluid. Fluid is also directed to the lymphatics

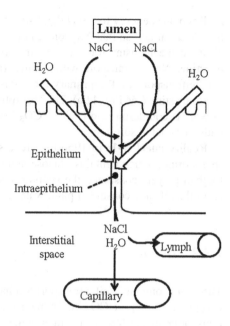

7.3 Intestinal Absorption

The absorption of fluid by the epithelial cells lining the villi occurs via a two-step process. First, solutes are absorbed followed by the *isosmotic absorption* of fluid. Hence, the solute and water are absorbed proportionately. The mechanisms for the absorption of solutes vary depending upon the location in the GI tract, e.g., jejunum, ileum or colon. In the absorbing state, the hydrostatic combined with the osmotic pressures in the intraepithelial space, interstitial space, and the capillaries favors the absorption of fluid (Fig. 7.2). In the secretory or nonabsorbing state, the high osmotic pressure in the lumen attracts fluid from the cytosol and interstitial space which results in secretion.

7.3.1 Jejunum

The apical borders of intestinal cells contain carrier molecules, which assist in the absorption of specific substances. The majority of Na^+ absorption occurs in the jejunum and is mediated by several Na^+-dependent cotransporters such as Na^+–monosaccharide (Na^+–glucose, Na^+–galactose), Na^+–amino acid, and Na^+–H^+ (see Figs. 4.9a, 6.6, and 6.7). The source of H^+ for Na^+–H^+ exchange comes from the conversion of CO_2 and H_2O in the presence of carbonic anhydrase to produce H^+ and HCO_3^- (see Fig. 4.9a). Na^+ cotransport with organic solutes and Na^+ movement through pores is driven by the concentration difference. The hydrolysis of

ATP provides energy to the Na^+/K^+ -ATPase pump located at the basal portion of the intestinal cell so that Na^+ ions can be pumped out of the cell. The presence of different mechanisms for Na^+–Cl^- transport varies over the length of the small intestine. Na^+ cotransport with solutes (amino acids and sugars) and Na^+–H^+ countertransport are the primary mechanisms for Na^+ absorption in the proximal small intestine (see Fig. 4.9a). The absorption of Cl^- involves cotransport with Na^+ as well as countertransport with HCO_3^- (see Fig. 4.9b). In the jejunum $NaHCO_3$ undergoes net absorption.

Reality check 7-1: In 1966 researchers at the University of Florida created a sports drink, which contains glucose and electrolytes. It was noted that when the football players consumed the sports drink, their hydration level was replenished more than if they consumed plain water in equal volumes. Why?

7.3.2   Ileum

The ileum contains similar transport mechanisms compared to the jejunum with the exception of a Cl^-–HCO_3^- exchanger located in the apical membrane and a Cl^- transporter in the basolateral membrane (see Fig. 4.9b). H^+ is secreted into the lumen of the ileum via the Na^+–H^+ exchanger. Additionally, HCO_3^- secretion occurs by the Cl^-–HCO_3^- exchanger. These mechanistic differences contribute to the net absorption of NaCl by the ileum compared to the net absorption of $NaHCO_3$ by the jejunum.

Patients who experience severe bouts of diarrhea lose large amounts of HCO_3^- (derived from salivary, pancreatic, and intestinal sources) compared to the loss of Cl^-. Therefore, these patients experience a hyperchloremic metabolic acidosis. In addition, patients with diarrhea lose K^+ in their stools resulting in hypokalemia.

7.3.3   Colon

Epithelial cells of the large intestine or colon primarily function to absorb NaCl and water that were not absorbed by the small intestine. These cells are very efficient in this regard because they contain channels for Na^+ absorption and K^+ secretion (see Fig. 4.10). In the colon, aldosterone induces the synthesis of Na^+ channels leading to the subsequent increase in Na^+ absorption and K^+ secretion. The increased Na^+ that enters into the intestinal cell is pumped into the capillaries in exchange for K^+ pumped by the Na^+–K^+ ATPase located in the basolateral membrane.

So how does this all fit together? Large amounts of Na^+, K^+, HCO_3^-, and Cl^- are absorbed in the small intestine and colon. Material that enters the duodenum undergoes rapid osmotic equilibration with plasma. Water enters hypertonic solutions while Na^+ and Cl^- leave hypertonic solutions. In contrast, water is absorbed from hypotonic solutions via the relatively permeable junctions between the epithelial cells of the proximal small intestine. Moving from the duodenum toward the colon, the luminal concentrations of Na^+ and Cl^- become lower than their plasma concentrations, whereas K^+ becomes higher than the plasma (Table 7.1). The Na^+ concentration in the duodenum is ~140 mEq/L and is similar to the plasma concentration. Cl^- is the major anion in the duodenal lumen. As the material in the small intestine moves toward the jejunum, the Na^+ concentration drops to 125 mEq/L in the ileum. Cl^- and HCO_3^- are both major anions in the ileum. In the colon, Na^+ concentration decreases to approximately 40 mEq/L, with the major anions being Cl^- and HCO_3^-. K^+ concentration increases from approximately 5 mEq/L in the duodenum to 80 mEq/L in the colon. Cl^- and HCO_3^- are the major anions in the colon. The absorption of Na^+ becomes more efficient as the material moves toward the distal gut due to the decreasing permeability of the epithelium and its prevention of absorbed ions undergoing back diffusion in the distal gut. The distal gut is the site of most effective Na^+ absorption. However, the conservation of Cl^- is greater and Cl^- is exchanged for HCO_3^- in the distal gut. As the volume of intestinal contents decreases the K^+ ions are passively absorbed. However, net K^+ secretion occurs in the colon. When patients experience diarrhea, they lose a significant amount of K^+ and HCO_3^- which results in a hypokalemic metabolic acidosis.

Reality check 7-2: Tropical Sprue is a malabsorption disorder characterized by blunting and effacement of the small intestinal villi. Why do these patients present with diarrhea?

7.3.4 Intestinal Fluid and Electrolyte Secretion

The epithelial cells of the crypts secrete electrolytes and fluid. Chloride ion channels are located on the apical membranes of the intestinal cells (Fig. 7.3). The basolateral membrane contains both a Na^+–K^+ ATPase and a Na^+–K^+–$2Cl^-$ cotransporter which brings in sodium, potassium, and chloride ions from the blood. Cl^- subsequently diffuses into the intestinal lumen via chloride ion channels (CFTR) in the apical membrane. Sodium ions follow chloride ion secretion passively and via a paracellular route. Water follows the secretion of sodium chloride into the lumen. Normally, the apical membrane Cl^- channels are closed. However, if certain neurotransmitters or hormones, e.g., acetylcholine (ACh) or vasoactive intestinal peptide (VIP), bind to the basolateral membrane receptors then the apical membrane Cl^- channels will open due to the activation of adenylyl cyclase and the generation of cAMP by the crypt cells. Cl^- secretion will occur in response to the opening of the Cl^- channels and Na^+ and water will follow Cl^- into the intestinal lumen.

Table 7.1 Luminal concentrations of Na$^+$, K$^+$, and Cl$^-$

Ion	Duodenum (mEq/L)	Ileum (mEq/L)	Colon (proximal) (mEq/L)	Plasma (mEq/L)
Na$^+$	140	125	40	140
K$^+$	5	23	80	4
Cl$^-$	100	90	30	100

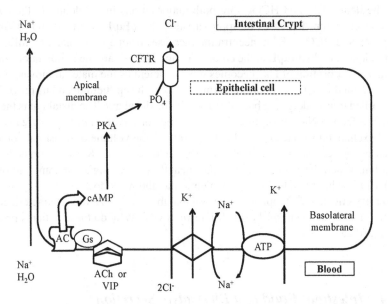

Fig. 7.3 Secretion of chloride by epithelial cells of intestinal crypts. Two Cl$^-$ enter the cell from the blood along with a Na$^+$ and K$^+$ ion. Na$^+$ is secreted to the blood in exchange for K$^+$ via the Na$^+$–K$^+$ pump (ATP). On the basolateral membrane either vasoactive intestinal peptide (VIP) or acetylcholine (Ach) can bind to its respective receptor, which interacts with Gs protein that in turn activates adenylyl cyclase (AC) to produce cAMP. The cAMP-dependent protein kinase A (PKA) opens the chloride channel (CFTR) allowing secretion of Cl$^-$, Na$^+$, and H$_2$O follow the Cl$^-$ passively via paracellular diffusion

7.3.5   Recall Points

- Absorption of solutes precedes isosmotic absorption of fluid.
- Different mechanisms for Na$^+$–Cl$^-$ absorption vary over the length of small intestine.
- Compared to the jejunum, the ileum also has an apical membrane Cl$^-$–HCO$_3^-$ exchanger and a basolateral membrane Cl$^-$ transporter.
- Aldosterone induces synthesis of Na$^+$ channels in the colon and subsequent Na$^+$ absorption and K$^+$ secretion.

7.4 Diarrheal Disorders

Diarrhea is arbitrarily defined as the passage of loose, watery bowel movements, generally more than three times per day, totaling 200 mL of stool per 24 h and is generally self-limited. When diarrhea lasts for 3 or more weeks, the condition is considered chronic. In underdeveloped countries, diarrhea is one of the top causes of death. The very young and the very old are most susceptible to the ravages of fluid and electrolyte disturbances caused by diarrhea. Some of the common causes of diarrhea include infections (due to viruses, bacteria, or parasites), food intolerances, artificial sweeteners, inflammatory bowel disorders, and medications (antibiotic associated, anticancer and antihypertensive agent induced). Travelers to foreign countries may develop diarrhea by consuming contaminated water or foodstuffs. Factitious diarrhea occurs when patients dilute their stools with liquids in order to dupe a healthcare provider. Such diarrhea is seen more commonly in patients seeking secondary gain or in those who have mental illness.

7.4.1 Osmotic Diarrhea

The major types of diarrheal disorders seen in clinical practice include osmotic, secretory, and reduction of the absorptive area of the intestines. An osmotic diarrhea results from an increase of osmotically active solute in the feces that elicits increased secretion of fluid into the intestinal lumen and hence the stool. Patients suffering from lactose intolerance cannot effectively hydrolyze lactose to glucose and galactose, resulting in an increase in osmotically active solutes in the intestinal lumen and resultant stool. Similarly, consuming excessive amounts of nonabsorbable artificial sweeteners, such as sorbitol and xylitol, can induce an osmotic diarrhea as well.

Fecal Osmolar Gap: Consider a sample of stool. In general, the osmolality of stool is close to that of serum (i.e., 290 mOsm/kg). Na^+ and K^+ are the two major cations present in stool. Normally, an equal number of anions must accompany cations present in the stool. Hence, doubling the sum of Na^+ and K^+ concentrations can account for both cations and anions in the stool sample. Therefore, the fecal osmolar gap $= 290 - [2(\text{stool } Na^+ + \text{stool } K^+)]$. The fecal osmolar gap represents the amount of unmeasured solutes in a stool sample. Patients with an osmotic diarrhea exhibit an elevated osmotic gap (>50 mOsm) due to the presence of additional unmeasured ions. Let us examine the following case. An elderly patient develops diarrhea after consuming excessive amounts of an antacid containing magnesium (Mg^{2+}). Measurement of his stool reveals: osmolality, 360 mOsm/kg; Na^+, 40 mmol/L; and K^+, 90 mmol/L (normal stool osmolality is 290 mOsm/kg; Na^+, 40 mmol/L; K^+, 90 mmol/L). The calculated fecal osmotic gap of this patient would be 360–260 mOsm $= 100$ mOsm. Hence, this patient has an osmotic diarrhea due to the presence of additional unmeasured Mg^{2+} in his stool.

Reality check 7-3: A patient undergoes a major surgical resection of both large and small intestines which results in the production of chronic diarrhea and hence loose watery stools. If you measure the osmolality of a stool sample from this patient, would you expect an increase, a decrease, or no change in the fecal osmotic gap?

Reality check 7-4: A university administrator presents to the GI clinic today complaining of chronic diarrhea. According to the patient and the chart she has had an extensive work up by outside gastroenterologists including endoscopies with biopsies, stools for ova and parasites, enteropathogens, inflammatory bowel disease, and endocrine disorders. All of her work-up has been normal. Upon eliciting a thorough dietary history, you discover that the patient consumes several diet sodas per day. You instruct the patient to stop drinking the diet sodas and record how many bouts of diarrhea she has per day. The patient returns to see you in 1 month and reports that her diarrhea has ceased. Based upon the physiological principles discussed in this chapter, what was the most probable cause of her diarrhea and how might you test your theory?

7.4.2   Secretory Diarrhea

Secretory diarrhea is caused by abnormal ion transport across the epithelial cells of the intestine that results in an increase in secretion, decrease in absorption, or a combination of both. Secretory diarrhea is caused by excessive secretion of fluid by crypt cells. Enteropathogenic bacteria such as toxigenic *E. coli* and *Vibrio cholerae* are major causative agents of secretory diarrhea. Basically, there is an overgrowth of pathogenic bacteria, and in the case of cholera, the cholera toxin crosses the apical membrane of the crypt cells (see Fig. 4.13b). Once the toxin enters the cell, the A subunit of the toxin undergoes detachment and moves across the cell until it reaches the basolateral membrane where it catalyzes adenosine diphosphate (ADP) ribosylation of the alpha$_s$ subunit of the G$_s$ protein which is coupled to adenylyl cyclase. Consequently, GTPase activity is inhibited and GTP cannot be converted back into GDP. Adenylyl cyclase is permanently activated when GTP remains permanently bound to the alpha$_s$ subunit. This modification results in cAMP levels remaining high and the Cl$^-$ channels remaining open. Na$^+$ and water secretions accompany the Cl$^-$ secretion. Due to the voluminous amount of fluid and electrolyte secretion, the absorptive capacity of the small and large intestine is overcome and the patient experiences severe diarrhea. Patients with a secretory diarrhea have a low osmotic gap (<50 mOsm/kg) because the secretions of cations and anions remain balanced.

7.4.3 Reduced Absorptive Area-Induced Diarrhea

Diarrhea induced by reduced absorptive surface area may result from the surgical resection of intestine or infiltration of the bowel wall resulting in a reduced area available for absorption of fluid and electrolytes. Examples of reduced absorptive surface area diarrhea include intestinal resection, infiltrative bowel diseases due to connective tissue disorders, ulceration, and inflammation.

Reality check 7-5: A patient with a long-standing history of mental illness is referred to the GI clinic for evaluation of chronic diarrhea. Colonoscopy and upper endoscopy with biopsies, stools for enteropathogens, parasites, HIV, thyroid disease, carcinoid syndrome were all nonrevealing. The patient turns in a stool sample which she collected at home. Laboratory evaluation is significant for a stool osmolality which is markedly lower than that of the plasma from a normal individual. In addition, the concentrations of sodium and potassium are markedly decreased. Based upon your understanding of the physiological principles discussed in this chapter, what do you think is responsible for these findings and how might you prove it?

7.4.4 Recall Points

Major Types of Diarrhea
- Osmotic
- Secretory
- Reduced absorptive surface area (due to surgery, inflammation, infiltration, ulceration)

Case in Point 7-1

Chief Complaint: A 20-year-old male presents to the student infirmary complaining of a 2-week history of diarrhea.

History: The patient is the president of the university outdoors club who recently returned from a 3-week camping trip to Colorado. The patient states that he drank water both from a stream and from a well. His other complaints include gaseousness, bloating, and nausea. The patient denies taking any medications, contact with ill people, or family history of GI disorders. He has no history of fever, vomiting, or hematochezia.

Physical Exam: On examination, the patient shows mild acute distress. His mucous membranes are slightly dry and he is not jaundiced. Lungs and heart exam are normal. The abdomen is soft, mildly distended, and without

(continued)

hepatosplenomegaly. Neurological, musculoskeletal, and skin exams are normal. The stool is negative for occult blood.

Labs:

Hb 14.2 g/dL [*N*: 13.8–17.2]	Hct 47 % [*N*: 41–52 %]
RBC 5.3 × 10^6 cells/μL [*N*: 4.2–5.5]	WBC 10.8 × 10^3 cells/μL [*N*: 6.8–13.3]
Platelets 275 × 10^9 cells/L [*N*: 164–351]	Albumin 3.2 g/dL [*N*: 3.5–5]
Sodium 145 mEq/L [*N*: 133–146]	Potassium 3.4 mEq/L [*N*: 3.7–5.2]
Chloride 110 mEq/L [*N*: 96–111]	Bicarbonate 23 mM [*N*: 22–29]

Stool Analysis: routine culture, ova and parasite testing revealed Giardia intestinalis trophozoites with Kohn stain. *Clostridium difficile* toxin is negative.

Assessment: On the basis of the history, physical exam, and lab findings what is the cause of this patient's acute diarrhea? How would you approach treating this patient?

Connecting-the-Dots 7-1

A 21-year-old man is brought to your Bangladesh medical mission infirmary because of massive diarrhea due to cholera. On physical examination, he appears acutely ill and in marked distress. Vital signs are significant for hypotension, tachycardia, and tachypnea. The patient skin is wrinkled with minimal turgor. His eyes are sunken, and he has dry mucous membranes. The abdominal exam is remarkable for a moderately distended, generally tender abdomen with increased bowel sounds. Laboratory tests are significant for severe metabolic acidosis, hyponatremia, and hypokalemia. The patient is excreting a massive amount of stool (more than 1 L/h). Measurement of the fecal osmotic gap was less than 50 mOsm/kg. What is the likely physiological cause of the patient's findings?

7.5 Summary Points

- Fluid secreted by the intestinal tract is 7 L per 24 h.
- Fluid consumed by the average person is 2 L per 24 h.
- Most (all but 100–200 mL) of the fluid is absorbed by the intestinal tract per 24 h.
- Diarrhea results from insufficient absorption of intestinal fluids.
- Folds of the mucosae (e.g., plicae circulares, villi, microvilli) greatly increase the absorptive surface area of the intestine.

- Absorption of intestinal fluids occurs at the level of the villi.
- Absorption of solutes precedes fluids.
- Crypt cells secrete electrolytes and fluids.
- Digestive enzymes are bound to the microvilli membranes.
- Material which enters the duodenum undergoes rapid osmotic equilibration with plasma.
- The majority of Na^+ absorption occurs in the jejunum.
- The jejunum contains several Na^+-dependent cotransporters (i.e., Na^+–glucose, Na^+–galactose, Na^+–amino acid and Na^+–H^+).
- The presence of different mechanisms for Na^+–Cl^- transport varies over the length of the intestine.
- Absorption of Cl^- involves cotransport with Na^+ and countertransport with HCO_3^-.
- Net absorption of HCO_3^- occurs in the jejunum.
- The apical membrane of the ileum contains a Cl^-–HCO_3^- exchanger and a basolateral membrane Cl^- transporter.
- Large bouts of diarrhea result in HCO_3^- loss and hyperchloremic metabolic acidosis.
- Diarrhea results in K^+ loss in the stools.
- Colonic epithelial cells contain channels for Na^+ absorption and K^+ secretion.
- Aldosterone induces synthesis of Na^+ channels, absorption of Na^+ and K^+ secretion.
- Absorption of Na^+ becomes more efficient as material moves distally in the gut because of decreasing permeability of the epithelium and prevention of ion back diffusion.
- Intestinal cell apical membranes contain Cl^- channels.
- Intestinal cell basolateral membranes contain a Na^+–K^+ ATPase and a Na^+–K^+–$2Cl^-$ cotransporter, which brings Na^+, K^+, and Cl^- into the cell from the blood.
- Binding of acetylcholine or VIP to its respective basolateral membrane receptor activates adenylyl cyclase resulting in an increase in activity of cAMP-dependent protein kinase and subsequent opening of Cl^- channels.
- Fecal osmolar gap represents the amount of unmeasured solute in stool.
- Osmotic diarrhea results from an increase of osmotically active solutes in stool.
- Secretory diarrhea is caused by increased secretion of fluids, decreased absorption of fluids, or both.
- The A subunit of the *Vibrio cholerae* toxin reaches the intestinal cell's basolateral membrane causing cAMP to remain high and hence the Cl^- channels remain open.
- Causes of reduced absorptive surface area-induced diarrhea include surgical resection of intestine, bypass, infiltrative, and ulcerative intestinal conditions.

7.6 Review Questions

7-1. A patient is excreting a large volume of diarrheal stool over the last 2 days. Based upon your understanding of intestinal fluid and electrolyte transport, which of the following findings in the patient's stool would you expect?

    A. Decrease in HCO_3^- concentration
    B. Decrease in K^+ concentration
    C. Increase in Cl^- concentration
    D. Increase in HCO_3^- concentration
    E. No change in the patient's stool HCO_3^- concentration

7-2. Several hours after consuming a 2 lb box of diabetic chocolate (sweetened with nonabsorbable sorbitol), you experience diarrhea. Which of the following is the most likely mechanism responsible for your diarrhea?

    A. Absence of osmotically active solutes in the stool attracting water into the lumen
    B. Excessive secretion of fluid by intestinal crypt cells
    C. Presence of osmotically active solutes in the stool attracting water into the lumen
    D. Reduced absorptive surface area-induced diarrhea

7-3. Which of the following best describes the fecal osmolar gap measurement for a patient with a secretory diarrhea?

    A. Elevated due to the decreased concentration of unmeasured solutes
    B. Elevated due to the increased concentration of unmeasured solutes
    C. Not elevated due to the increased concentration of unmeasured solutes
    D. Not elevated due to the isosmotic concentration of solutes

7-4. A patient with diarrhea has Crohn's disease limited to her terminal ileum and characterized by transmural infiltration of the intestinal wall. Which of the following is the most likely cause of this patient's diarrhea?

    A. Excessive use of laxatives as a treatment for the Crohn's disease
    B. Osmotic diarrhea
    C. Reduced absorptive area-induced diarrhea
    D. Secretory diarrhea

7-5. An elderly woman took several extra doses of milk of magnesia for her constipation. She subsequently developed watery diarrhea. Her fecal osmolar gap was 150 mOsm. Which of the following best explains the most likely cause of her diarrhea?

    A. Osmotic diarrhea due to decreased Mg^{2+}
    B. Osmotic diarrhea due to increased Mg^{2+}
    C. Secretory diarrhea due to decreased Mg^{2+}
    D. Secretory diarrhea due to increased Mg^{2+}

7.7 Answer to Case in Point

Case in Point 7-1: The cause of this patient's diarrhea is a microscopic parasite called *Giardia lamblia*. *Giardia* is found on the surfaces of soil, food, and water. It is transmitted via fecal-oral contamination. The exact mechanisms of *Giardia* pathogenesis which leads to diarrhea and intestinal malabsorption are not completely understood. It has been speculated that attachment of trophozoites to the brush border could produce a mechanical irritation or mucosal injury. Metronidazole is the treatment of choice for giardiasis.

7.8 Answer to Connecting-the-Dots

Connecting-the-Dots 7-1: *Vibrio cholerae* produces a toxin which results in a secretory diarrhea. The massive amounts of fluid and electrolytes (especially Na^+, K^+, HCO_3^-) account for this patient's signs and symptoms of severe dehydration, metabolic acidosis, hyponatremia, and hypokalemia. Because the secretions of cations and anions are balanced, the fecal osmotic gap is low (less than 50 mOsm/kg). Treatment with World Health Organization (WHO) oral rehydration solution (water, glucose, sodium, potassium, and citrate) relies upon the coupled transport of sodium and glucose which will allow the intestinal cells to absorb salt and water more effectively.

7.9 Answers to Reality Checks

Reality check 7-1: The sport drink contained glucose and electrolytes. Water absorption from the small intestine can be enhanced by the presence of Na^+ and glucose (in certain concentrations) because of the cotransporters found in the intestinal membranes. The Na^+ and glucose will be actively transported into the intestinal cell, and H_2O will passively diffuse into the intercellular spaces via the tight junctions. Hence, the football players absorbed water more effectively and could play harder.

Reality check 7-2: Patients with Tropical Sprue develop a flattening of the small intestinal villi probably due to an infectious agent. Because these patients suffer from a loss of small intestinal absorptive area, they develop diarrhea due to a lack of fluid and electrolyte absorption. After a course of antibiotics, the villi return to their finger-like projecting state and increase the absorptive surface for fluids and electrolytes.

Reality check 7-3: Patients with marked reductions in intestinal absorptive surface area fail to absorb foodstuffs and their digestive products effectively which will result in an increase in osmotically active solutes in the stool and an increased osmotic gap compared to normal individual.

Reality check 7-4: Diet sodas contain nonabsorbable sugars which attract water into the intestinal lumen and create an osmotic diarrhea. By removing the offending agent (the diet sodas) the patient's symptoms subside. If you challenge the patient by allowing her to consume diet sodas and her diarrhea returns, then your suspicion that the diet sodas induced an osmotic diarrhea would be corroborated.

Reality check 7-5: Factitious diarrhea represents the intentional dilution of a stool sample by a patient in order to dupe a healthcare provider or another individual. A simple way to determine if a sample is representative of factitious diarrhea would be to collect another sample under observation and recheck the stool osmolality and electrolytes. If the second sample resulted in normal values, then the first sample was probably diluted with water or another substance. Factitious diarrhea occurs more commonly in patients with mental illness.

7.10   Answers to Review Questions

7-1. **D**. Patient with large volume diarrhea would excrete an increased amount of HCO_3^- as well as K^+. Hence, these patients would develop a hyperchloremic hypokalemic metabolic acidosis.

7-2. **C**. Sorbitol is a nonabsorbable sweetener which is an osmotically active solute. Hence, more water will be attracted into the intestinal lumen, resulting in an osmotic diarrhea.

7-3. **C**. Patients with a secretory diarrhea secrete a proportionate amount of solutes. Hence, their fecal osmolar gap is not elevated.

7-4. **D**. Crohn's disease patients with involvement of the terminal ileum will experience an interruption of the enterohepatic circulation of bile salts. These patients will have an increased amount of bile salts in the colon which will result in a bile salt-induced secretory diarrhea.

7-5. **B**. Mg^{2+} is an osmotically active solute which will produce an osmotic diarrhea. You would expect this patient to have an increased fecal osmolar gap.

Suggested Reading

Costanzo LS. Gastrointestinal physiology (Chapter 8). In: Physiology. 4th ed. Philadelphia: Saunders-Elsevier; 2010. p. 327–78.

Johnson LR. Fluid and electrolyte absorption (Chapter 12). In: Gastrointestinal physiology. 8th ed. Philadelphia: Elsevier-Mosby; 2014. p. 128–38.

Kibble JD, Halsey CR. Gastrointestinal physiology (Chapter 7). In: The big picture: medical physiology. New York: McGraw Hill; 2009. p. 259–306.

Chapter 8
Gastrointestinal Manometry: Tales of the Intrepid Transducer

8.1 Introduction

Motility is literally the engine that drives the GI tract. In the absence of motility, digestion and absorption would be exceedingly difficult. Gastroenterologists are frequently consulted to diagnose and assist in the management of patients with upper or lower GI tract motility disorders. In this chapter, representative dysmotility cases are presented. Through the interpretation of physiological data obtained by the manometric (motility) transducer, the reader is provided the opportunity to use recently acquired knowledge to solve clinical problems.

8.2 Refractory Gastroesophageal Reflux Disease

Gastroesophageal reflux (GER) is a normal physiological process which individuals experience multiple times per day and is not a disease. GER is generally asymptomatic. In contrast, *gastroesophageal reflux disease* (GERD) occurs as a result of the inability of normal antireflux mechanisms to guard against abnormal amounts and frequent episodes of gastroesophageal reflux. GERD patients frequently complain of heartburn symptoms. Mechanisms of GERD include most commonly transient lower esophageal sphincter (LES) relaxations, swallow-induced LES relaxations, hypotensive LES pressure, hiatus hernia-induced compromise of LES function, decreased esophageal acid clearance, insufficient salivary gland secretion, increased gastric acid secretion, and delayed gastric emptying. Several conditions are associated with GERD. In pregnancy, circulating estrogen and progesterone may lower LES pressure. In patients with scleroderma, smooth muscle fibrosis lowers LES pressure and amplitude of peristalsis. Finally those with Zollinger–Ellison syndrome exhibit hypersecretion and increased volume of gastric acid.

E. Trowers and M. Tischler, *Gastrointestinal Physiology*,
DOI 10.1007/978-3-319-07164-0_8, © Springer International Publishing Switzerland 2014

Upon endoscopic examination, the majority of GERD patients will not exhibit obvious mucosal injury. However, some GERD patients have erosions, ulcerations, strictures, and/or mucosal changes of Barrett's esophagus. Patients with GERD may also complain of aspiration-related pulmonary and vocal cord symptoms. Surgery is generally reserved for patients with severe complications of obstruction or aspiration-related problems. On the other hand, some patients may opt for a nonpharmacologic approach due to difficulties in procuring medications or for compliance issues.

Sample Case 8-1: Jack McDuff is a 57-year-old used car salesman who had frequent bouts of severe heartburn provoked by lying down, bending over to tie his shoes, or eating a greasy meal. He complained of heartburn and occasional difficulty on swallowing solid food, diminution of appetite, 5 lb weight loss (over 2 months), chronic cough, frequent bouts of pharyngitis, laryngitis, sinusitis, and exacerbation of asthma. Mr. McDuff reported that he experienced control of his symptoms on twice-daily proton pump inhibitor (PPI) treatment. On physical examination, Mr. McDuff had a flare of heartburn upon assuming the supine position. Otherwise, his examination was unremarkable. Upper endoscopy revealed a large hiatus hernia with mild diffuse gastritis. A barium esophagogram revealed a nonreducible large hiatus hernia (Fig. 8.1). Esophageal manometry revealed effective esophageal peristalsis, but decreased LES pressure (Fig. 8.2). Twenty-four hour pH testing was indicative of GERD. Gastric emptying studies were within normal limits. The patient stated that he wanted surgery because of drug expense and a fear of unknown long-term medication side effects.

Reality Check 8-1: Based upon your analysis of Mr. McDuff's history, physical examination, and lab results, why do you think that he was diagnosed with GERD?

Reality Check 8-2: Why is surgery a reasonable option for Mr. McDuff?

Reality Check 8-3: You are a surgeon planning a fundoplication (wrap procedure to reinforce the LES) for a patient whose esophageal manometric study shows decreased contractions in the esophageal body and poor clearance of a test food bolus. Should you make your wrap either tighter or less tight and what is your reasoning for this choice?

8.2.1 Recall Points

- GERD is generally caused by transient relaxation of the LES and failure of normal antireflux mechanisms.
- Surgical indications for refractory GERD patients include:
  - Failure of medical therapy
  - Risk of severe pulmonary or vocal cord injury
  - Noncompliance with maintenance medications
  - Cost concerns regarding chronic medication expenses

Fig. 8.1 Line drawing of
an esophagram showing a
hiatus hernia

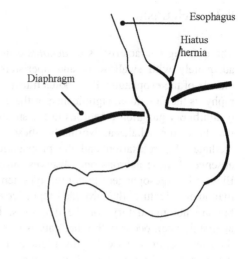

Fig. 8.2 Esophageal
manometry revealed
effective esophageal
peristalsis, but decreased
lower esophageal sphincter
(LES) pressure (*dotted line*,
hypotensive LES)

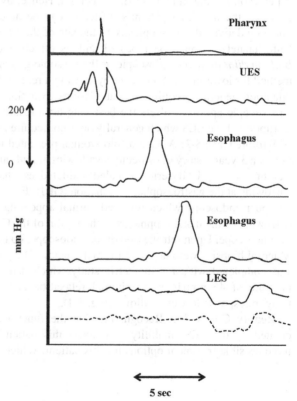

8.3 Achalasia

The defining characteristics of *achalasia* include the failure of the LES to relax adequately with swallowing and aperistalsis or hypoperistalsis in the smooth muscle of the esophagus. Poor bolus transit, as detected by fluoroscopy or scintigraphy, is the functional significance of these manometric findings. The destruction of inhibitory ganglionic neurons in the smooth muscle esophagus is the pathological basis for achalasia. Normally, these intramural myenteric plexus neurons mediate LES relaxation and the propagation rate of peristalsis. Hence, in the absence of these neurons one observes impaired LES relaxation and aperistalsis. Elevated intraesophageal pressure, hypertensive LES, or isobaric waveforms are manometric features that provide supportive evidence for the diagnosis of achalasia but are not mandatory for the diagnosis. It is important to note that because aperistalsis can occur with other causes of esophageal dysmotility disorders (e.g., diabetes, collagen vascular disorders and GERD), the diagnosis of achalasia depends on finding-impaired LES relaxation. Hence, by decreasing LES sphincter pressure, the achalasia patient's difficulty can be ameliorated. Botulinum toxin injection delivered endoscopically to the site of the LES is an effective treatment. Unfortunately, it must be repeated and its effectiveness diminishes over time. *Balloon dilatation* via endoscopic or fluoroscopic guidance is another noninvasive method for lowering LES pressure by causing a rent in the LES. However, balloon dilatation generally requires repeat sessions over time. Surgical myotomy via a laparoscopic approach offers the best long-term results because it is a controlled disruption of the LES which generally does not require repeat surgical intervention.

Sample Case 8-2: A 33-year-old woman presented to the GI clinic for evaluation of a 3-year history of difficulty swallowing liquids and solids, as well as a 20-lb weight loss. An UGI series revealed a dilated esophagus with a "bird's beak" narrowing at the gastroesophageal junction (GEJ) (Fig. 8.3). The patient underwent an upper endoscopy which revealed normal appearing esophageal mucosa and a narrowing of the distal esophagus in the region of the GEJ that allowed passage of the endoscope. Upon retroflexion of the endoscope, no tumor was noted at the GEJ. Mucosal biopsies were negative for malignancy. The patient's diagnostic work-up was completed with a manometric study which demonstrated an elevated LES pressure of 45 mmHg with minimal relaxation and an aperistaltic esophageal body in response to wet swallows (Fig. 8.4).

Reality Check 8-4: Recognizing that the functional obstruction at the GEJ created by the LES' inability to relax is this patient's major problem suggest three possible treatment options for this patient. Which option is best and why?

Fig. 8.3 Line drawing of an UGI esophagram. (**a**) Normal. (**b**) A dilated esophagus with a "bird's beak" narrowing at gastroesophageal junction in an achalasia patient

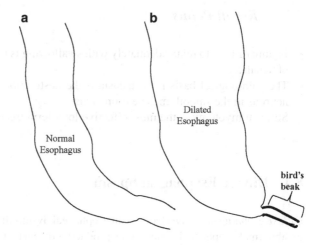

Fig. 8.4 Esophageal manometric tracing in an achalasia patient demonstrating an elevated LES (*dotted line*, hypertensive LES) of 45 mmHg with minimal relaxation and aperistaltic esophageal body in response to a wet swallow

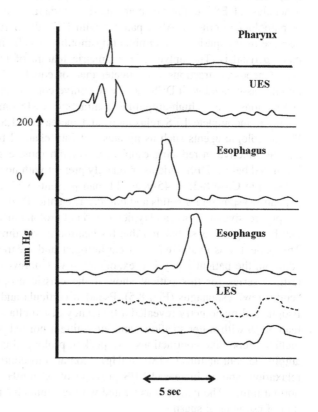

8.3.1 Recall Points

- Failure of LES to relax adequately with swallowing is the defining characteristic of achalasia.
- The pathological basis for achalasia is the destruction of inhibitory ganglionic neurons in the smooth muscle esophagus.
- Surgical myotomy is the most effective long-term treatment for achalasia.

8.4 Diffuse Esophageal Spasm

Diffuse esophageal spasm (DES) is an esophageal dysmotility, which is characterized by abnormal esophageal contractions producing dysphagia and/or chest pain. Selective, intermittent dysfunction of the myenteric plexus is the likely etiology. Compared to achalasia, DES is defined by manometric criteria rather than by clinical, functional, or pathological criteria. Also, patients with DES differ from those with achalasia because they experience intermittent dysmotility which alternates with normal primary peristalsis. The universal manometric feature of DES is the occurrence of simultaneous contractions with greater than or equal to 30 % of swallows. Other findings associated with DES include repetitive contractions (>2 peaks), prolonged contractions (>6 s), high-amplitude contractions (>180 mmHg), spontaneous contractions, incomplete LES relaxation, and increased LES pressure (>40 mmHg). Pharmacologic agents such as nitrates, calcium channel blockers, and hydralazine can be effective in reducing esophageal smooth muscle spasm in small trials. As illustrated below, DES patients frequently present with noncardiac chest pain.

Sample Case 8-3: A 45-year-old man presents with a 4-year history of chest pain and dysphagia for solids and liquids. The patient's dysphagia was intermittent, nonprogressive in nature, and typically did not prolong mealtime. The patient stated that his weight was stable and that his heartburn was diminished by taking a PPI. The patient was evaluated by a cardiologist and cleared of cardiac disease. In addition, the patient's physical examination was unrevealing. An upper gastrointestinal series for this patient showed the classic esophagogram findings of a "corkscrew" esophagus (Fig. 8.5). Pseudodiverticula and curling were not noted. Esophageal manometry revealed a frequency of simultaneous contractions greater than 30 % with water swallows and intermittent normal peristalsis. Other findings included repetitive contractions (>2 peaks), prolonged contractions (>6 s), high-amplitude contractions (>180 mmHg), spontaneous contractions, incomplete LES relaxation, and an increased LES pressure of 65 mmHg. Endoscopy was within normal limits. The patient was treated with calcium channel blockers with resolution of esophageal spasms.

Sample Case 8-4: Mrs. Dower, a 54-year-old woman, presents to the Emergency Department complaining of a squeezing retrosternal chest pain radiating to the neck, jaw, arms, and back. In addition, the patient tells you that she frequently experiences dysphagia for both solids and liquids. She took some of her husband's

Fig. 8.5 Line drawing of an UGI esophagram. (**a**) Normal. (**b**) Diffuse esophageal spasm depicting "cork screw" esophagus

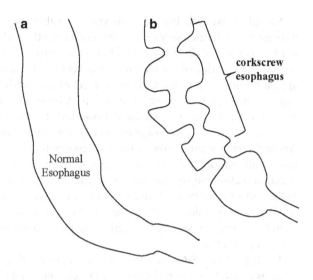

nitroglycerine tablets and experienced significant relief. You are concerned that the patient has an esophageal motility disorder, e.g., achalasia or DES versus a cardiac origin for chest pain.

Reality Check 8-5: For Mrs. Dower, which diagnosis do you think is more important to evaluate initially and why?

8.4.1 Recall Points

- DES is an esophageal dysmotility associated with abnormal esophageal contractions causing dysphagia and/or chest pain.
- DES is associated with greater than or equal to 30 % of nonperistaltic (simultaneous) contractions.
- DES is an intermittent phenomenon with periods of normal peristalsis.

8.5 Hirschsprung's Disease

Hirschsprung's disease or *congenital megacolon* is caused by the absence of ganglion cells from the myenteric and submucosal plexuses, as noted on full-thickness or suction (mucosal–submucosal) biopsy specimen of the rectum. Contents proximal to the lesion fail to enter the unrelaxed aganglionic segment. The most characteristic functional abnormality of *aganglionosis* is a failure of the internal anal sphincter (IAS) to relax. The defect occurs in 1 out of 5,000 live births and is familial in some cases. Hirschsprung's disease should be suspected shortly after birth when an infant presents with abdominal distention and passes little meconium.

Sample Case 8-5: Imagine that you are a third-year medical student rotating through the pediatrics service and you encounter the following patient. A 10-year-old boy is referred for evaluation of chronic constipation and abdominal bloating. Digital examination of the rectum causes retained fecal material to gush forth with apparent relief of symptoms. However, relief is short-lived with the return of the signs of incomplete intestinal obstruction. A barium enema X-ray film reveals the characteristic transition from the narrowed, distal rectum to the dilated proximal colon (Fig. 8.6). A proctosigmoidoscopy revealed a normal but empty rectum. Anorectal manometry showed the IAS contracting instead of relaxing following balloon distention of the rectum. The external sphincter function remains normal. Mucosal suction biopsy does not reveal ganglion cells. Surgical consultation results in the performance of a full-thickness biopsy of the rectum at 4 cm proximal to the pectinate line and documents the absence of ganglion cells. The youngster subsequently undergoes surgical resection of the aganglionic segment without any residual problems.

Reality Check 8-6: Based upon your understanding of the role of myenteric neurons in the functioning of smooth muscle sphincters, how can you account for the narrow aganglionic segment noted on the patient's barium enema X-ray?

8.5.1 Recall Points

- Hallmark of Hirschsprung's disease is the absence of ganglion cells from the myenteric and submucosal plexuses.
- Characteristic functional abnormality of aganglionosis is failure of internal sphincters to relax following rectal distention.
- Barium enema X-ray confirms diagnosis if characteristic transition from the narrowed, distal rectum or rectosigmoid to the dilated proximal colon is seen.

8.6 Fecal Incontinence

Fecal incontinence is the expulsion of feces against one's wishes. This can be a very embarrassing problem and may have a great impact upon a patient's social interaction with others. Under normal circumstances, the anal canal is 3–4 cm long and forms the distal outlet of the gut. It normally remains closed by tonic contractions of the surrounding muscles. The *internal anal sphincter* (IAS) is formed from the circular smooth muscle layer of the rectum and is under autonomic control. The IAS is responsible for the majority of resting anal canal tone. The *external anal sphincter* (EAS) is a surrounding sleeve of striated muscle that blends into the puborectalis and levator ani muscles proximally and extends to just below the IAS margin distally. The EAS is a voluntary muscle, which is innervated by the pudendal nerve and contributes approximately 30 % to the resting anal tone. The

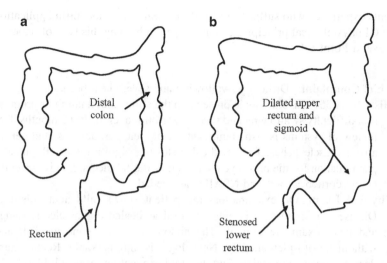

Fig. 8.6 Line drawing of barium enema. (**a**) Normal. (**b**) Characteristic transition from the stenosed, lower rectum to the dilated proximal colon in a Hirschsprung's disease patient

EAS exerts a significant role in maintaining continence by contracting reflexly during sudden rectal distention or increased abdominal pressure. If the EAS is voluntarily contracted, the normal resting tone of the anal canal doubles.

The causes of fecal incontinence include but are not limited to the following: diarrhea, anal pathology (carcinoma, rectal prolapse, perianal infections), rectal pathology (carcinoma, proctitis), neurological diseases (stroke, dementia, multiple sclerosis), peripheral nervous system disorders (diabetes, cauda equina lesions), and trauma (childbirth injuries, descending perineum, old age).

Clinical evaluation of the incontinent patient should include a thorough history to assess the acuity, frequency, and degree of debility associated with the symptoms as well as history of trauma, neurological disease, infection, or other risk factors, e.g., diabetes, rectal prolapse, and anorectal infections. Physical exam should include inspection of the perianal area to look for lesions and digital examination to assess for sphincter tone as well as for anorectal angle, fecal impaction, and rectal prolapse.

The extent of clinical testing to evaluate the mechanisms of fecal incontinence depends upon the patient's clinical presentation and the availability of local expertise. Inspection of the distal colon by anoscopy and sigmoidoscopy is a minimum requirement. Inflammatory conditions and tumors may be noted and appropriate investigation can be instituted. Anorectal manometry can be performed to assess sphincter function by measuring resting and maximal squeeze pressures of the anal canal using miniaturized transducers, perfused catheters, and balloons. Anorectal ultrasound can be performed to examine the structural integrity of the IAS and EAS.

Defecography evaluates defecation by video fluoroscopic imaging. The following Connecting-the-Dots illustrates the significant social ramifications which patients experience who suffer from fecal incontinence. Thoughtful application of basic GI physiological principles can assist you in helping this type of patient.

Case in Point 8-1

Chief Complaint: Difficulty swallowing and severe heartburn.

History: A 35-year-old female presents to the clinic complaining of progressive difficulty swallowing and severe heartburn over the last 2 months. Her review of systems is also significant for nausea, gaseousness, and generalized muscle aches. Past medical history is significant for Raynaud's phenomenon for the past 3 years as well as digital ulcers. She is currently taking corticosteroids and NSAIDS as needed.

Physical Exam: On examination, the patient shows mild acute distress. Diffuse fibrosis of skin is noted as well as healed digital ulcers. Lungs and heart exam are normal. The abdomen is soft, nondistended, and without hepatosplenomegaly. Neurologic is unremarkable. Rectal exam does not reveal any masses and the stool is negative for occult blood.

Labs:

Hb 10.2 g/dL [N: 14.7–18.6]	Hct 37 % [N: 43–56 %]
RBC 3.5 × 10^6 cells/μL [N: 4.2–5.5]	WBC 10.6 × 10^3 cells/μL [N: 6.8–13.3]
Platelets 175 × 10^9 cells/L [N: 150–450]	Albumin 4.0 g/dL [N: 3.5–5]
Sodium 137 mEq/L [N: 133–146]	Potassium 3.6 mEq/L [N: 3.7–5.2]
Chloride 111 mEq/L [N: 96–111]	Bicarbonate 24 mM [N: 22–29]

Serology tests reveal a high-titer ANA by indirect immunofluorescence, with a titer of >1:640 in a centromere pattern. Barium swallow X-ray revealed a dilated esophagus (in the lower two-third region) with hypotensive peristaltic contractions and poor esophageal clearance. Upper endoscopy revealed erosive esophagitis. Manometry revealed decreased resting pressure and very low amplitude simultaneous contractions in the distal esophagus. LES pressure was hypotensive.

Assessment: On the basis of the history, physical exam, and lab findings what is the cause of this patient's difficulty with swallowing and heartburn? How would you approach treating this patient?

Connecting-the-Dots 8-1

A 33-year-old otherwise healthy woman presents with a 1-year history of episodic fecal incontinence. The patient states that she has restricted her professional and social activities out of fear and embarrassment. The patient states that vigorous exercise routinely precipitates fecal incontinence. Hence, she wears incontinence pads for protection against soiling her clothes. The

(continued)

patient's surgical history is significant for the repair of a third-degree perineal laceration involving the vagina, IAS, and EAS, and which occurred during the vaginal delivery of her daughter 9 years ago. Otherwise, her past medical history is unremarkable and she has no neurological complaints. Physical examination reveals decreased resting sphincter tone and reduced voluntary squeeze. Given this patient's past surgical history of obstetrical trauma, why would the performance of anorectal manometry and anorectal ultrasound be useful?

8.6.1 Recall Points

- Fecal incontinence is the loss of feces against one's wishes.
- Most patients with fecal incontinence can be treated with dietary modifications, pharmacologic interventions, and/or biofeedback training.
- The extent of clinical testing depends upon the patient's clinical presentation and the availability of local expertise.

8.7 Summary Points

- GERD may be caused by transient relaxation of LES, hypotensive LES, swallow-induced LES relaxation, hiatus hernia-induced compromise of LES, poor esophageal acid clearance, decreased salivary and esophageal gland secretion, as well as increased gastric acid secretion.
- Antireflux surgery is generally reserved for GERD patients who are refractory to medical treatment or at risk for pulmonary/vocal cord complications. Compliance with medications and financial issues may influence surgical indications.
- The defining characteristic of achalasia is the failure of the LES to relax adequately with swallowing.
- Achalasia is caused by the destruction of inhibitory ganglions in the smooth muscle of the esophagus.
- The "bird's beak" narrowing of the distal esophagus with upstream dilation is a classic radiographic sign seen on a barium esophagram.
- Surgical myotomy is the most effective long-term achalasia treatment.
- DES is an esophageal dysmotility which occurs intermittently and is associated with greater than or equal to 30 % of simultaneous contractions which are nonperistaltic.
- DES is associated with chest pain, high amplitude contractions, increased LES pressure, and incomplete LES relaxation.

- Hirschsprung's disease is caused by the absence of ganglion cells from the myenteric and submucosal plexuses in the rectum. Other areas of the intestine may also be involved.
- Inability of the IAS to relax is the most characteristic functional abnormality of Hirschsprung's disease.
- Barium enema X-ray confirms the diagnosis of Hirschsprung's if the characteristic transition from the narrowed, distal rectum or rectosigmoid to dilated proximal colon is noted.
- Fecal incontinence is due to the expulsion of feces against one's wishes.
- Common causes of fecal incontinence include trauma, infection, neurological disorders.
- The extent of clinical testing to evaluate the mechanisms of fecal incontinence depends upon the patient's presentation and the availability of local expertise.

8.8   Review Questions

8-1. Of the following mechanisms, which is the most frequent cause of GERD?

    A. Decreased esophageal gland secretion
    B. Decreased salivary secretions
    C. Sliding hiatus hernia
    D. Transient LES relaxation

8-2. Of the following features, which is the signature characteristic of achalasia?

    A. Elevated intraesophageal pressure
    B. Failure of LES to relax with swallowing
    C. Hypertensive LES
    D. Poor bolus transit

8-3. Which of the following is the key distinguishing feature between DES and achalasia?

    A. Chest pain
    B. High amplitude contractions
    C. Incomplete relaxation of LES with swallowing
    D. Intermittent normal peristalsis

8-4. Hirschsprung's disease has a similar etiologic mechanism compared to another motility disorder. Which of the following disorders fits this description?

    A. Achalasia
    B. DES
    C. Fecal incontinence
    D. Refractory GERD

8-5. Which of the following tests should all patients with fecal incontinence undergo?

    A. Anorectic manometry
    B. Anorectic ultrasound
    C. Defecography
    D. Sigmoidoscopy

8.9 Answer to Case in Point

Case in Point 8-1: This scleroderma patient has severe ineffective esophageal motility and an incompetent LES due to the infiltration of fibrotic tissue. Essentially, her esophagus is likened to a rigid pipe. Consequently her peristaltic waves are markedly diminished. Her compromised LES allows for free reflux of gastric acid that produces heartburn. Treatment should be directed at treating the underlying scleroderma as well as vigorous antireflux measures such as maximum doses of PPIs, head of the bed elevation and dietary modifications.

8.10 Answer to Connecting-the-Dots

Connecting-the-Dots 8-1: Most patients with fecal incontinence will respond to dietary measures and pharmacologic agents directed toward the underlying cause. However, a subgroup of patients will be refractory to medical therapy and will be surgical candidates. Anorectal manometry can assess the strength and functionality of the IAS and EAS. Anorectal ultrasound can be used to image the IAS and EAS to see if they are damaged and amenable to surgical repair.

8.11 Answers to Reality Checks

Reality Check 8-1: A good history is sufficient to make the diagnosis of GERD in most cases. Mr. McDuff complains of heartburn triggered by large fatty meals and exacerbated by assuming a supine position and by activities which increase intra-abdominal pressure, e.g., bending over to tie his shoes. In addition, he states that the pain is relieved by PPIs. Upper GI series revealed a large nonreducible hiatus hernia which may compromise the proper functioning of the LES. In addition, 24 h pH monitoring documented significant reflux of gastric acid.

    Reality Check 8-2: Most GERD patients can be successfully treated with life style changes (avoidance of large fatty or spicy meals especially within 2 h of going to bed), antireflux measures such as elevating the head of the bed, avoidance of alcohol, nicotine, and acidic beverages. Mr. McDuff was a candidate for antireflux surgery (fundoplication) because he had a large nonreducible hiatus hernia which mechanically compromised his LES. In addition, he had symptoms compatible with aspiration involving his nasopharynx and lungs. Further indications for surgery included the fact that he could not afford long-term maintenance PPI therapy and was afraid of taking medication for prolonged periods of time.

Reality Check 8-3: Patients with decreased esophageal body contractions have more difficulty clearing food boluses. If you make a tight wrap in the region of the LES this would further impede the clearance of a food bolus. Hence, you should probably make your wrap less tight compared to your normal wrap.

Reality Check 8-4: One option for relieving the functional obstruction caused by the LES' inability to relax might be a pharmacologic approach. Smooth muscle relaxants (e.g., calcium-channel blockers and nitrates) might help to decrease the LES pressure. Unfortunately, the efficacy of this treatment is short-lived and inconsistent. Botulinum toxin could be injected into the region of the LES to cause paralysis of the sphincter. This approach initially produces good results, but generally must be repeated at 6–12-month intervals. A problem with this approach is that it can cause fibrosis at the injection site thus complicating future surgical procedures. A second option would encompass physically stretching and/or disrupting the LES. Balloon dilatation causing an esophageal myotomy produces very good results initially, but repeat dilatation is often required. In addition, the risk of perforation increases with the larger sized balloons. The third option, laparoscopic surgical myotomy, is a minimally invasive technique which yields excellent long-term relief, but this should only be considered for patients who are good surgical candidates and who have not been helped by the above-mentioned noninvasive options. In the extreme case, surgical resection of the esophagus would obviate the problem caused by the functional obstruction of the GEJ.

Reality Check 8-5: A cardiac origin for chest pain should be ruled out initially prior to attributing the patient's chest pain to an esophageal motility disorder. This is an extremely important point to keep in mind. Coronary artery disease is more common than esophageal motility disorders presenting as chest pain. In addition, coronary artery disease is associated with a greater morbidity and mortality rate compared to esophageal motility disorders, e.g., achalasia or DES.

Reality Check 8-6: The ganglion cells are responsible for the ability of the smooth muscles to relax and move bowel contents forward. Hence, in the absence of the ganglion cells in the involved segment, the bowel will be contracted which forms an obstruction to the passage of stool. Surgical resection of the diseased segment will remove the obstruction and allow for the passage of stools.

8.12 Answers to Review Questions

8-1. **D**. Transient relaxation of the LES is the most common cause of GERD symptoms, followed by other causes of LES compromise, e.g., hypotensive LES.

8-2. **B**. Incomplete relaxation of the LES is the hall mark of achalasia. Aperistalsis and/or hypoperistalsis may also be present but is not required to make the diagnosis.

8-3. **C**. The key distinguishing feature between DES and achalasia is incomplete relaxation of LES with swallowing.

8-4. **A**. Hirschsprung's disease or congenital megacolon is due to the absence of ganglion cells from the myenteric and submucosal plexuses. Achalasia is also due to aganglionosis.

8-5. **D**. All patients with fecal incontinence should undergo sigmoidoscopy to assess for masses or inflammation as a cause of sphincter compromise.

Suggested Reading

Janson LW, Tischler ME. The digestive system (Chapter 11). In: The big picture: medical biochemistry. New York: McGraw Hill; 2012. p. 149–66.

Johnson LR. Motility of the large intestine (Chapter 6). In: Gastrointestinal physiology. 8th ed. Philadelphia: Elsevier-Mosby; 2014. p. 47–53.

Kahrilas PJ, Pandolfino JE. Esophageal motor function (Chapter 9). In: Yamada T, Alpers DH, Kalloo AN, Kaplowitz N, Owyang C, Powell DW, editors. Textbook of gastroenterology. 5th ed. Oxford, UK: Wiley-Blackwell; 2009.

Richter JE. Gastroesophageal reflux disease (Chapter 32). In: Yamada T, Alpers DH, Kalloo AN, Kaplowitz N, Owyang C, Powell DW, editors. Textbook of gastroenterology. 5th ed. Oxford, UK: Wiley-Blackwell; 2009.

Appendix A

Table A.1 Diseases affecting GI tract and organs involved with digestion

Name	Description	Signs and symptoms	Treatment
Oral cavity and salivary			
Aphthous stomatitis (canker sores)	Common ulcers caused by various irritations such as biting your cheek or burning your mouth. They are not contagious. Three types are minor (80 %; 2–4 mm diameter), major (~21 cm diameter), and herpetiform ulcers.	Minor ulcers cause minimal symptoms. Major ulcers are more painful requiring longer to heal. Herpetiform ulcers mainly in females begin with vesiculation and progress to multiple, minute often extremely painful ulcers.	Primarily topical corticosteroids. Topical tetracycline may reduce severity as well as mouth rinses. Anti-inflammatory agents may help as well as oral vitamin B_{12}.
Herpetic stomatitis (cold sores)	Viral infection causing vesicles and painful shallow ulcers with inflammation. A contagious disease caused by herpes simplex virus (HSV).	Oral blisters on the tongue, cheeks, palate, or gums. Food intake decreases. Swallowing difficulty (dysphagia), drooling, fever, and swollen gums.	Treated with acyclovir. Mostly a liquid diet of nonacidic drinks recommended. Numbing medicine helps with severe pain.
Necrotizing sialometaplasia	Benign ulcerative lesion usually on the posterior portion of the hard palate. From necrosis of minor salivary glands as a result of trauma and possibly transient local ischemia.	Ulcers (single, bilateral, or multiple) are deep and necrotic with a flat edge. Can be up to 3 cm in diameter. Condition may involve mild pain or paresthesia. Typically resolves in 6–10 weeks.	No treatment recommended though a biopsy is recommended to rule out a malignancy.
Sialolithiasis (salivary stones)	Calcified mass forms in a salivary gland. Increased calcium or Sjögren's syndrome may be causal factors.	Pain and swelling of affected gland that worsens with increased salivary flow. Inflammation and/or infection may occur.	Removal of calcified mass. Rarely the submandibular gland may be removed. Lithotripsy more effective with parotid than submandibular stones.

(continued)

Table A.1 (continued)

Name	Description	Signs and symptoms	Treatment
Sjögren's syndrome	Autoimmune disease in which antibodies produced against salivary glands. Results in decreased secretions (e.g., saliva and tears). Inflammation of the glands leads to decreased saliva production. May be an inherited disorder with 90 % of patients female.	Mouth dryness (xerostomia), dysphagia, salivary stones, dental decay, extraglandular problems such as joint pain, arthritis, fatigue.	No cure. Excess fluid consumption for dry mouth, saliva stimulant medications, artificial saliva preparations.
Thrush	Yeast infection of the mucus membrane lining mouth and tongue. Usually appears when immune system is weak. Important factors include poor health, elderly, very young, HIV infection or AIDS, chemotherapy, steroid medications.	Whitish, velvety sores; underlying red tissue that may bleed.	Mild cases: consuming yogurt. Diabetics: controlling blood glucose. Antifungal mouthwash or lozenges. HIV/AIDS: antifungal medications.
Esophagus			
Achalasia	Affects the ability of the esophagus to move food to the stomach caused by the failure of the lower esophageal sphincter (LES) to sufficiently relax due to damage or degeneration of ganglion cells innervating the esophagus.	Most common is dysphagia, as well as regurgitation, chest pain that may increase after eating, coughing, heartburn, difficulty burping, or unintentional weight loss.	Goal is to reduce pressure at the LSE including Botox injection to relax the muscles, drugs (nitrates or calcium channel blockers) to relax the LES, pneumatic bag dilation, and/or surgery to decrease the pressure or dilation of the esophagus where narrowing occurs.
Barrett's esophagus	Stomach acid leaking backwards through the LES resulting in change of esophageal lining to specialized columnar cells. Lining of esophagus damaged by stomach acid often associated with GERD (see below).	Symptoms are those of acid reflux disease. Endoscopy shows red velvety mucosa (Barrett's) contrasting with pale pink esophageal squamous mucosa.	Treatment of acid reflux with antacids, histamine H2 receptor blockers, or proton pump inhibitors. Severe dysplasia may require endoscopic ablation or surgery to remove precancerous tissue.
Boerhaave syndrome	Spontaneous transmural perforation of the esophagus most commonly due to concurrent negative intrathoracic pressure coupled with increased intraesophageal pressure usually associated with emesis.	Present with retching and vomiting leading to intense retrosternal and upper abdominal pain followed by rapid development of painful swallowing, tachypnea, dyspnea, cyanosis, fever, and shock.	Associated with high morbidity and mortality so lack of therapy can be fatal. Because of its rarity little guidance for treatment and depends on the location and size of the perforation as well as other factors. Thoracic perforations require surgery. Cervical

(continued)

Table A.1 (continued)

Name	Description	Signs and symptoms	Treatment
			perforations are manageable without surgery.
Candida	Most common fungus infecting the esophagus. Most often found in diabetics, HIV-infected patients or those with malignancies affecting the hematological system.	Painful swallowing localized to a discrete retrosternal area. Endoscopy reveals white mucosal plaque-like lesions with cultured biopsy showing Candida.	Therapeutic antifungal agents including polyenes, azoles, and echinocandins.
Esophageal varices	Swollen blood vessels of the esophagus usually associated with serious liver disease (e.g., cirrhosis).	Symptoms only occur if the vessels leak or burst leading to vomiting of blood, fainting, dark-colored stool, or lightheadedness.	Treatment focuses on decreasing likelihood of bleeding using beta-blockers to reduce blood pressure, losing weight, and avoiding alcohol. Variceal band ligation used to stop the bleeding.
Gastroesophageal reflux disease (GERD)	Stomach acid backs up into the esophagus due to a relaxed (due to stomach distension) or weakened LES. GERD results when the acid reflux causes significant symptoms or injury to the esophagus.	Patients exhibit heartburn that starts in the chest and may spread to the throat along with acid taste in the throat. Less frequently: stomach pain, difficult or painful swallowing, persistent laryngitis or sore throat, chronic cough, regurgitation, dental disease, pneumonia, chronic sinusitis, or awakening with a choking sensation.	Mild acid reflux treated with dietary change, antacids, or histamine antagonists. More serious symptoms require proton pump inhibitors and surgery in the most severe cases.
Mallory–Weiss syndrome	Longitudinal mucosal lacerations in the distal esophagus (also proximal stomach) associated with forceful retching. Usually secondary to suddenly increased intra-abdominal pressure precipitated by vomiting, straining, coughing, convulsions, blunt abdominal trauma amongst others.	Primarily acute GI bleeding accompanied by epigastric pain or pain in the back. Bleeding occurs if the tear involves the esophageal venous or arterial plexus. Nonbloody vomiting or retching may precede bloody vomiting.	Many (40–70 %) patients require transfusions though most tears heal spontaneously. Endoscopic therapy treats bleeding lacerations. Injection of epinephrine to diminish arterial flow or electrocoagulation may be used. Patients also prescribed a proton pump inhibitor though benefit in preventing rebleeding is unclear.
Plummer–Vinson syndrome	Occurs in patients with chronic iron deficiency anemia. Formation of esophageal webs that are thin mucosal folds protruding into the lumen to partially block the esophagus. The exact cause is unknown.	Patients have difficulty swallowing and weakness. This rare disorder has been linked to esophageal and throat cancers more often in women.	Iron supplements may improve swallowing problems. Endoscopic laser division or resection with end-to-end anastomosis to widen the esophagus.
Reflux esophagitis	Excessive stomach acid reflux combined with impaired clearance of the refluxate in the esophagus. Pathophysiology includes transient LES relaxation, hypotensive LES, or	Difficult and/or painful swallowing, heartburn associated with acid reflux, sore throat or hoarseness, mouth sores, nausea, vomiting, indigestion, chest pain, and	When due to infection an antibiotic is required. Proton pump inhibitors reduced stomach acid production. When induced by medications

(continued)

Table A.1 (continued)

Name	Description	Signs and symptoms	Treatment
	disruption of the gastro-esophageal junction associated with hiatal hernia.	bad breath are all associated symptoms.	(e.g., anti-inflammatory) a change is needed.
Zenker's diverticulum (pharyngo-esophageal diverticulum)	An outpouching of the pharynx mucosa just above the upper sphincter of the esophagus. Excessive pressure of the lower pharynx causes the wall to balloon out. Causes include uncoordinated swallowing and impaired sphincter muscle relaxation.	Though asymptomatic the diverticulum may lead to swallowing difficulty, sense of a lump in the neck, regurgitation, halitosis, infection of the pharyngeal areas (due to stuck food), and gurgling noise when swallowing.	None needed when small and asymptomatic. Larger diverticula may require resection. Endoscopic stapling to close the diverticulum is used as a nonsurgical approach. Laser treatment may be less effective than stapling.

Stomach

Name	Description	Signs and symptoms	Treatment
Acute gastritis	Usually transient mucosal inflammatory process. Associated with use of aspirin and other NSAIDs, alcohol consumption, heavy smoking, chemotherapy, etc. May also be caused by *H. pylori* infection (see below). Damage from disruption of the mucosal layer followed by increased acid and decreased bicarbonate secretion with reduced mucosal blood flow.	Gnawing or burning epigastric distress that may be accompanied by nausea or vomiting. Eating may improve or worsen the pain.	When cause by *H. pylori* infection, the bacteria require eradiation and proton pump inhibitors may also be needed.
Autoimmune gastritis	Development of autoantibodies to gastric parietal cells and acid producing enzyme (H^+–K^+ ATPase) (90 %) and/or intrinsic factor (60 %). Associated with other autoimmune diseases (Hashimoto's thyroiditis; Addison's disease).	Progressive atrophy of the stomach with loss of parietal cells diminishing acid production and causing secondary hypergastrinemia. Loss of intrinsic factor prevents vitamin B_{12} absorption causing pernicious anemia.	Pernicious anemia as a complication must be treated by vitamin B_{12} replacement. If related to *H. pylori* infection it must be eradicated.
Chronic gastritis	Long-term changes leading to mucosal atrophy and intestinal metaplasia. Etiology includes infection, immunologic response (see autoimmune gastritis), toxic (e.g., alcohol, smoking), chemical (reflux of duodenal	Asymptomatic though can have upper abdominal discomfort, nausea, and vomiting. Additionally there can be bloating, indigestion, hiccups, loss of appetite, vomiting blood, or black, tarry stools.	Treatment depends on cause as discussed above for *H. pylori* infection and complications of autoimmune gastritis. Drugs that cause gastritis must be discontinued. Neutralization or decreased production of stomach acid can

(continued)

Table A.1 (continued)

Name	Description	Signs and symptoms	Treatment
	secretions), and motor or mechanical (e.g., obstruction).		eliminate symptoms and promote healing.
Cyclic vomiting syndrome	Episodes or cycles of severe nausea and vomiting lasting for hours to days Alternate with intervals without symptoms. Occurs in all age groups and may be related to occurrence of migraine headaches.	Phases include: (a) symptom-free interval between episodes; (b) prodrome—episode of nausea and vomiting about to begin; (c) nausea and vomiting with inability to eat, drink, or take medicines without vomiting; paleness; drowsiness; (d) recovery when nausea and vomiting stop; healthy color, appetite, energy return.	Patients learn to control symptoms. Advised to get rest and take medications that prevent vomiting, stop one in progress, speed up recovery, or relieve symptoms. During vomiting, stay in bed; sleep in a dark, quiet room. Severe nausea and vomiting may require hospitalization and IV fluids to prevent dehydration. Sometimes, can stop an episode by using drugs for nausea or ibuprofen for pain. Drugs that calm the stomach by lowering acid may help. Drinking water and replacing lost electrolytes are important.
Helicobacter pylori gastritis	Infection damages the mucosal layer. Colonizes the surface of gastric epithelial cells. Bacteria produce urease that hydrolyzes urea to ammonia and bicarbonate creating an alkali environment. May elicit a local immune response. See other descriptions of gastritis above.	Same as with other descriptions of gastritis above.	The bacteria require eradiation and proton pump inhibitors may also be needed.
Menetrier's disease	Hyperplastic hypersecretory gastropathy associated with enlarged gastric mucosal folds accompanied by increased total stomach weight. Profound hyperplasia of the surface mucous cells with glandular atrophy. An increased risk for stomach cancer.	Protein loss, parietal cell atrophy, and an increase in mucous cells. Patients exhibit epigastric pain after a meal. Common to have weight loss, cachexia, peripheral edema, ascites, and anemia symptoms secondary to blood loss.	Gastrectomy and a high-protein diet are the only treatments. Antacids may relieve pain. Part or all of the stomach may need to be removed if disease is severe. The monoclonal antibody cetuximab has been used.
Peptic ulcer disease	Disruption of surface mucosa extending beyond muscularis mucosae. Ulcers are chronic, often solitary lesions mostly in the stomach and proximal duodenum. Lifetime likelihood of developing peptic ulcer is ~10 % for American men; ~4 % for American women. Approx 70 % of patients with gastric ulcers not	Burning pain aggravated by stomach acid contacting ulcerated area. Pain may be felt from navel to the breastbone, worsen with empty stomach, flare at night, temporarily relieved by foods that buffer stomach acid, or disappear and then return for a few days or weeks. There may be vomiting of blood, black or tarry stools, nausea or	Eradication of *H. Pylori*. Proton pump inhibitors or histamine H2 antagonists.

(continued)

Table A.1 (continued)

Name	Description	Signs and symptoms	Treatment
	attributed to NSAID are infected with *H. pylori*.	vomiting, unexplained weight loss, or appetite changes.	
Pernicious anemia	Autoimmune destruction of parietal cells or weakened stomach lining resulting in hypochlorhydria; sometimes autoantibodies to intrinsic factor. Average age of diagnosis is 60. Most common in those of Scandinavian or northern European heritage. Prior diagnosis of other autoimmune disorders increases the risk.	Symptoms may be absent or mild but can include diarrhea, fatigue, loss of appetite, pallor, swollen/red tongue, bleeding gums, shortness of breath during exercise.	Increase plasma B_{12} by injections monthly or more often depending on severity because of loss of intrinsic factor from parietal cells.
Pancreas			
Acute pancreatitis	Sudden inflammation that is reversible over a short period of time. Most common causes include alcohol consumption, gallstones, a variety of metabolic disorders, abdominal trauma, penetrating ulcers, certain drugs, and a variety of infectious agents.	Gradual or sudden upper abdominal pain that may radiate to the back. May be accompanied by nausea, vomiting, diarrhea, loss of appetite, chills, tachycardia, respiratory distress, and/or peritonitis.	Depends on severity. Correction of predisposing factors causing acute attack and reduce inflammation. Pain control, bowel rest, and nutritional support. Endoscopic retrograde cholangiopancreatography within 72 h of attack of gallstone pancreatitis may reduce morbidity and mortality.
Chronic pancreatitis	Most commonly after episode of acute pancreatitis with ongoing inflammation that does not heal or improve. Prolonged alcohol use accounts for almost half the cases. Other causes include gallstones, hereditary disorders, cystic fibrosis, high plasma triglycerides, and certain drugs.	Damage due to alcohol may take years to manifest followed by sudden development of severe symptoms including pain and loss of function resulting in abnormal digestion and blood glucose homeostasis. Other symptoms may be similar to that of acute pancreatitis (see above).	Hospitalization for management of the pain, hydration, and nutritional support. When continuing to lose weight may require nasogastric intubation feeding. Synthetic pancreatic enzymes used to aid digestion. Consumption of alcohol and smoking must be avoided.
Cystic fibrosis	Inherited disease with buildup of thick, sticky mucus in lungs and digestive tract, especially the pancreas. Thick mucus from defective transport of Cl^- and Na^+ across epithelium of the affected tissue. Thick mucus in pancreatic ducts blocks secretion of digestive enzymes that accumulate and attack	Symptoms associated with digestion problems. Failure to process dietary triglycerides reduces absorption of fat and fat soluble vitamins (i.e., A, D, E, K). Vitamin deficiencies lead to problems relevant to their specific functions. Failure to secrete digestive enzymes leads also to	There is no cure. Treatment to ease symptoms and reduce complications. Pancreatic enzyme and fat soluble vitamins supplements. Feeding tube may be used at night to boost overall daily caloric intake. If chronic pancreatitis develops treatment as described above is used.

(continued)

Table A.1 (continued)

Name	Description	Signs and symptoms	Treatment
	pancreatic cells with irreversible damage leading to chronic pancreatitis.	malnutrition with poor growth and development due to reduced caloric intake.	
Zollinger–Ellison syndrome	Associated with increased gastrin production often resulting from small pancreatic tumor, a gastrinoma that may appear in the small intestine. The high and uncontrolled gastrin production increases stomach acid secretion. A rare disease with diagnosis between ages 30 and 50.	Excess gastric acid secretion often can cause peptic ulcers. Patients exhibit abdominal pain, diarrhea, and may vomit blood depending on the severity of the ulcers.	Excess acid production treated with proton pump inhibitors. Inhibitors also help heal peptic ulcers and relieve pain and diarrhea. If the tumor has not spread to other organs, then a single gastrinoma may be excised.

Gallbladder, liver, and hepatic bile ducts

Name	Description	Signs and symptoms	Treatment
Acute acalculus cholecystitis	Acute necroinflammatory disease resulting from reduced blood flow (ischemia) through the cystic artery. No gallstones are present. Usually occurs in critically ill patients after major nonbiliary surgery, severe trauma or burns, multiorgan system failure, sepsis, prolonged intravenous hyperalimentation, or postpartum. Less commonly occurs in outpatients with vasculitis or AIDS.	There may be no localizing signs or symptoms and may not be recognized early. Because it is often subtle with a gradual onset diagnosis can be difficult.	Immediate intervention is essential because of a high risk of gallbladder perforation. For those who can tolerate surgery, cholecystectomy is performed.
Acute calculus cholecystitis	Most common complication of gallstones results from chemical irritation and inflammation that occurs when the gallbladder neck or cystic duct become obstructed. Recurrent attacks are common.	Right upper quadrant or epigastric pain. Patients may have mild fever, anorexia, tachycardia, diaphoresis, nausea, and/or vomiting. Jaundice suggests an obstruction of the common bile duct.	Those with progressively severe symptoms require immediate surgery; up to ~25 % of patients. However attacks usually resolve in 24 h though may last up to a week.
Acute cholecystitis	Sudden inflammation of the gallbladder mostly (90 %) caused by gallstones. Bile, trapped in the gallbladder, irritates the gallbladder and produces pressure. These events can lead to infection and perforation.	Severe abdominal pain that can be sharp, cramping, or dull. It may be steady and may spread to the back or below the right shoulder blade.	Patients given fluids and antibiotics to treat infection. Cholecystectomy is usually required.
Biliary atresia	Complete obstruction of bile flow due to destruction or absence of some or all of	Children normal at birth but rapidly develop neonatal jaundice and acholic	The Kasai surgical procedure connects the liver to the small intestine generally

(continued)

Table A.1 (continued)

Name	Description	Signs and symptoms	Treatment
	the extrahepatic bile ducts. Bile is trapped and damages the liver. Most common cause of liver disease in early childhood.	stools. Associated symptoms include dark urine, enlarged spleen, and slow growth with slow or no weight gain.	prior to 8 weeks of age. Usually a liver transplant is still needed.
Cholangitis	Bacterial infection of the bile ducts that is termed "ascending" if it enters the intrahepatic ducts. "Suppurative" form refers to pus-producing condition extending into the hepatic parenchyma causing abscesses. Usually caused by gram-negative rod bacteria.	Patients may have fever, chills, abdominal pain, and/or jaundice.	Quick diagnosis and treatment are critical. Antibiotics are administered. Endoscopic retrograde cholangiopancreatography or other surgery may be performed especially in very ill patients or those rapidly worsening.
Choledocholithiasis	Stones in the hepatic or common bile duct that may result in cholangitis (see above), obstructive jaundice, or pancreatitis. Most stones pass into the duodenum.	Asymptomatic unless stone blocks the common bile duct. Symptoms then occur as described for specific types of cholecystitis.	Goal to alleviate blockage by ERCP and/or surgery to remove the stones or a sphincterotomy that cuts the muscle in the common bile duct to allow passage of stones.
Cholelithias	Formation of gallstones either cholesterol (75–80 %) or pigmented (bilirubin-containing) in up to 20 % of adults in developed countries. Risk factors include ethnicity, age, sex, obesity, metabolic errors, and family history. Risk factors for pigmented stones include hemolytic syndromes or biliary tract infections.	Most patients (80 %) are asymptomatic. Symptoms are associated with stones lodging in a duct causing a blockage. Symptoms can then occur as described for specific types of cholecystitis.	Treatment depends on the disease stage. Once symptoms appear, cholecystectomy is usually indicated. Other treatments can reduce the risk of further stone formation such as oral bile salt therapy, contact dissolution, and extracorporeal shockwave lithotripsy.
Chronic cholecystitis	Occurs when swelling and irritation of the organ continues. May be caused by repeated acute attacks due to gallstones in the gallbladder. Walls of the gallbladder thicken and the organ may shrink. As the disease continues, the gallbladder's ability to concentrate, store, and release bile decreases.	Symptoms specific to the chronic disease are unclear and likely are largely the same as those of acute disease.	Laparoscopic cholecystectomy is the most common treatment. When the patient is too ill for surgery, oral medication may be used to dissolve the gallstones though this may take up to 2 years and stones may return.
Primary biliary cirrhosis	An autoimmune disease of the liver associated with slow progressive destruction of small bile ducts of the liver. Intralobular ducts are affected early in	Approximately 50–60 % asymptomatic at diagnosis. Patients may exhibit fatigue, pruritus, jaundice, xanthomas (especially near the eyes), and	Complications requiring therapy include pruritis, malabsorption of dietary fat, fat soluble vitamin deficiencies, hypothyroidism, iron deficiency

(continued)

Table A.1 (continued)

Name	Description	Signs and symptoms	Treatment
	the disease. Damage to these ducts causes bile accumulation that damages the liver. It is more prevalent in females (9:1).	usual symptoms of cirrhosis and portal hypertension (i.e., ascites, splenomegaly, esophageal varices, hepatic encephalopathy).	anemia, and liver failure. Treating the immunologic attack has been less successful.
Primary sclerosing cholangitis	A chronic progressive disorder that leads to cholestasis and hepatic failure. The etiology leading to the inflammation and narrowing of intra- and extrahepatic biliary ducts is unknown.	Asymptomatic or may have fatigue and pruritis. May also exhibit splenomegaly, jaundice, hepatomegaly, or skin abrasions. Radiography reveals abnormal bile ducts with wall thickening, strictures, and dilations.	Immunosuppressive and anti-inflammatory drug therapy without evidence of success. Endoscopic therapy may help those with a dominant extrahepatic biliary stricture. When liver disease is advanced, transplantation is likely. Other surgical approaches include biliary reconstruction. In some patients with ulcerative colitis protocolectomy may be necessary due to increased colorectal cancer risk.

Intestine (small and large)

Name	Description	Signs and symptoms	Treatment
Abetalipoproteinemia (Bassen–Kornzweig syndrome)	An inherited disorder associated with an inability to produce chylomicrons and very low density lipoprotein (VLDL) due to deficiency of either the B apoprotein (B48, chylomicrons; B100, VLDL) or of the microsomal triglyceride transfer protein (MTTP). Disease manifests in the first few months of life.	Impaired absorption of dietary lipids and fat soluble vitamins leads to severe hypolipidemia especially of serum triglycerides. Failure to thrive and usually diarrhea, steatorrhea, and star-shaped red blood cells (acanthocytosis). Other symptoms from fat soluble vitamin deficiencies: vitamin E; impaired nervous system function (ataxia); vitamin D-dependent rickets; and vitamin K-easy bruising.	Diet low in long-chain triglycerides and cholesterol essential. Substitution with medium-chain triglycerides in the diet beneficial as they do not use chylomicrons for absorption. Dietary lipids need to include essential fatty acids such as in safflower oil. Supplementation with fat soluble vitamins and minerals.
Angiodysplasia	Caused by aging and degeneration of blood vessels resulting in their becoming swollen and fragile primarily in the colon. Swelling becomes so severe that a small passage develops between a small artery and vein, an arteriovenous fistula.	Elderly patients exhibit weakness, fatigue, and shortness of breath due to anemia. Bleeding directly into the colon may or may not occur and when it does the stool contains bright, red blood. Patients do not exhibit pain.	If bleeding then cause and rate of blood loss needs to be determined. Fluid replacement and blood products as the situation dictates. Bleeding may cease without treatment. Treatment may include angiography to block the vessel that is bleeding. Other drugs, e.g., thalidomide and estrogens, have been tried per orally

(continued)

Table A.1 (continued)

Name	Description	Signs and symptoms	Treatment
			in nonemergent cases. If cauterization or drugs are unsuccessful then hemicolectomy vs. total colectomy may be needed.
Celiac disease (celiac sprue)	Patients have a gluten-sensitive enteropathy. Glutens are a portion of proteins in certain grains to which they have an autoimmune reaction.	The autoimmune response destroys villi affecting digestion and absorption of all macronutrients. Symptoms relate to broad malabsorption including vitamin deficiencies. These include to varying extents digestive problems, severe skin rash, iron deficiency anemia, musculoskeletal issues, growth problems and failure to thrive, seizures, nerve damage and low calcium causing tingling, aphthous ulcers, or missed menstrual periods.	Gluten-free diet must be adhered to that excludes wheat, rye, and barley as grains or flour. In more severe cases oats must also be avoided but for mild cases can be consumed in small amounts. Patients must be advised that some medications contain gluten. Breads and pastas may be made from potato, rice, soy, or bean flour. Unprocessed meats, fish, fruits, and vegetables can complete the diet.
Cholera	*Vibrio cholerae* produces a toxin that leads to constantly active protein kinase A, which phosphorylates chloride channels that remain open. Allows chloride efflux to the lumen accompanied by paracellular movement of sodium and water.	Severe diarrhea, nausea and vomiting. Resulting dehydration accompanied by irritability, lethargy, sunken eyes, dry mouth, extreme thirst, dry and shriveled skin, little or no urine output, low blood pressure, and an irregular heartbeat.	Replace lost fluids and electrolytes using a simple rehydration solution; without rehydration, approximately half the people die. Most helped by oral rehydration alone, but those severely dehydrated may need IV fluids. Antibiotics are not a necessary treatment, but some (doxycycline or azithromycin) may reduce amount and duration of cholera-related diarrhea. Zinc supplements may decrease and shorten duration of diarrhea in children.
Clostridium difficile infection	Bacterial infection that causes diarrhea and potentially bacterial colitis. Prolonged use of antibiotics increases the risk of contracting infection especially in the elderly.	Watery diarrhea (at least three bowel movements per day for 2 or more days), fever, loss of appetite, nausea and abdominal pain, or tenderness.	Ideally stop using antibiotic that triggered infection but this is not always possible. Mild symptoms treated with metronidazole or alternatively vancomycin; fidaxomycin, a new antibiotic that appears equivalent to

(continued)

Table A.1 (continued)

Name	Description	Signs and symptoms	Treatment
			vancomycin but much more expensive. Never use antidiarrheal drugs as slowing an inflamed colon may cause a severe complication, toxic megacolon.
Crohn's disease	Inflammatory bowel disease that can affect any area of the GI tract from the mouth to the anus. Most common sites are ileum and colon. Inflammation may be confined to the bowel wall, leading to scarring, or inflammation may spread through the bowel wall (fistula).	Mild to severe and include diarrhea, abdominal pain, cramping, ulcers, reduced appetite, weight loss, and bloody stool. Less frequently patients exhibit fever, fatigue, arthritis, eye inflammation, mouth sores, skin disorders, inflammation of the liver and/or bile ducts, delayed growth and sexual development in children.	No cure so treatment focuses on relieving symptoms and to bring about remission.
Dysentery	Inflammatory disorder of the intestine, especially of the colon, that is a type of gastroenteritis. Results in severe bloody diarrhea often containing mucus with blood and accompanied by fever, abdominal pain, and rectal tenesmus (feeling of incomplete defecation). Can be caused by any kind of infection.	Mild symptoms consist of stomach pains and frequent passage of stool or diarrhea. Symptoms appear after 1–3 days and disappear by 1 week. Frequency of urge to defecate, volume of liquid feces passed, and presence of mucus, pus, and blood depends on the causal pathogen. Temporary lactose intolerance can occur. Severe abdominal pain, fever, shock, and delirium can all be symptoms. In extreme cases, patients complain of nausea, abdominal pain, and frequent watery, foul-smelling diarrhea, accompanied by mucus, blood, rectal pain, and fever. Vomiting, rapid weight loss, and generalized muscle aches sometimes also occur.	As with cholera (above) replace lost fluids and electrolytes using a simple rehydration solution. With severe dehydration may also need IV fluids. May be necessary to administer combination of drugs, including an amebicidal drug, to kill the parasite if due to amebiasis, or an antibiotic to treat any bacterial infection.
Escherichia coli infection	One of the most frequent causes of bacterial infections including cholecystitis (see above), cholangitis (see above), and traveler's diarrhea. The gastroenteritis	Time between infection and developing symptoms usually 24–72 h. Sudden, severe, and often bloody diarrhea the most common symptom. Other symptoms include fever,	Recovery usually without specific treatment within a few days with avoidance of dehydration. In general, antibiotics should not be given as the bacteria can lose

(continued)

Table A.1 (continued)

Name	Description	Signs and symptoms	Treatment
	involves inflammation—bacterial colitis.	gas, appetite loss, cramps, and rarely vomiting. Severe infection may include easy bruising, pale sin, red or bloody urine, and reduced urinary output.	releasing toxins that could cause hemolytic uremic syndrome especially in children. In the case of severe infection, antibiotics are needed.
Familial chloride diarrhea	An inherited disorder caused by excessive chloride secretion into the intestinal lumen.	Associated with large, watery stools containing an excess of chloride. Individuals have intrauterine (pre-birth) and lifelong diarrhea and infants with the condition are often premature. Excessive diarrhea causes electrolyte and water deficits, leading to volume depletion, renal potassium wasting, hyperreninemia, hyperaldosteronism, and sometimes nephropathy.	No cure so treatment focuses on the individual symptoms of the condition typically including oral supplements of sodium and potassium chloride.
Giardiasis	A parasitic disease caused by *Giardia lamblia*. A common cause of gastroenteritis affecting 200 million people worldwide.	Loss of appetite, diarrhea, blood in urine, stomach cramps, bloating, excessive gas last 1–2 weeks after infection.	Infection usually resolves itself. For persistent symptoms one of several drugs can be used.
Hartnup disease	Autosomal recessive defect in sodium-dependent transport protein for uncharged amino acids in the intestine. Poor absorption of uncharged amino acids many of which are essential including tryptophan; branched-chain amino acids; methionine; phenylalanine; histidine; threonine. Tryptophan required to make nicotinic acid a B vitamin, low nicotinic acid can cause pellagra that can lead to dermatitis, diarrhea, dementia, and even death.	Symptoms usually start in infancy, affecting mainly the brain and skin to include failure to thrive, mental retardation, short stature, headaches, altered gait (ataxia), tremor, fainting, irregular eye movements (nystagmus), and increased sun sensitivity. Psychiatric problems (anxiety, mood changes, delusions, and hallucinations) may also occur.	Treatment usually via a diet high in neutral amino acids, sunblock and/or sun avoidance and, when needed, daily intake of nicotinamide and sunblock. A period of poor nutrition usually precedes symptoms outbreaks and attacks.
Hirschsprung's disease	Congenital condition associated with blockage of the large intestine. Ganglion cells missing from part of the bowel prevent peristalsis with intestinal contents accumulating behind the blockage. Accounts for 25 % of newborn intestinal	Lack of meconium passed after birth; bowel movement difficulty; infrequent, explosive stools; poor feeding; low weight gain; watery diarrhea; jaundice; vomiting.	Serial rectal irrigation relieves pressure in bowel prior to surgery; abnormal section of colon surgically removed.

(continued)

Table A.1 (continued)

Name	Description	Signs and symptoms	Treatment
	blockage. Males affected five times more than females.		
Irritable bowel syndrome (spastic colon)	A chronic GI disorder that lacks a definitive organic cause. Decreased receptive accommodation in the proximal stomach is felt to play a role. Affects ~55 million in the USA, mostly women.	Symptoms include chronic abdominal pain, bloating, and altered bowel habits.	Dietary changes, exercise, and/or medications help with symptoms.
Ischemic colitis	Reduced blood flow to part of the colon as a result of narrowed or blocked arteries. Insufficient blood flow limits oxygen delivery to cells in the colon causing pain and cell damage. Can affect any part of the colon. Patients usually over age 60.	Pain usually on the left side of the abdomen along with cramping or tenderness. Stool contains bright red- or maroon-colored blood. Diarrhea and an urgency to move bowels.	Depends on the severity of the disease. In mild cases symptoms diminish in 2–3 days. Recommendations include antibiotics to avoid infection, IV fluids if dehydrated, and avoiding medications that can further constrict blood vessels.
Lactose intolerance	Inability to digest dietary lactose into glucose and galactose because of deficiency of the brush border enzyme lactase. Most common in the Black, Asian, Hispanic, and Native American populations.	Colonic bacteria process the lactose producing gas accompanied by osmotic diarrhea (see below), bloating, and vomiting.	Avoid lactose in the diet by limiting the intake of milk and milk products.
Meckel diverticulum	Congenital problem of a pouch on the wall of the lower part of the intestine. The parietal cell containing tissue is left over from the fetal digestive tract and is similar to tissue of the stomach.	Usually asymptomatic but can cause pain in the abdomen ranging from mild to severe, and blood in the stool.	In the case of bleeding, surgery may be needed to remove the portion of the small intestine containing the diverticulum. Iron supplements may be needed to correct anemia.
Microscopic colitis	Inflammation of the colon. Examination of colon tissue microscopically to identify [hence the name]. Types include collagenous colitis, thick layer of collagen develops in the colon or lymphocytic colitis, increased white blood cells in colonic tissue.	Persistent watery diarrhea along with abdominal pain or cramps, nausea, weight loss, and fecal incontinence.	When necessary begin with dietary change and medications. A low fat, low fiber diet and discontinuing medications that cause symptoms. Medications used may include antidiarrheal, bile salt sequestrant, steroids or anti-inflammatory, or immune suppressants.
Necrotizing enterocolitis	Acute inflammatory disease with death of the lining of the intestinal wall primarily in the terminal ileum or ascending colon. Specific cause is unknown and likely there are variable causes. Most	Abdominal distension, bloody stool, diarrhea, intolerance to feeding, lethargy, temperature instability, and vomiting are all potential symptoms. Death rate close to 25 %.	Feeding is stopped. Gas pressure relieved by a tube into the stomach. IV nutrition replaces oral. Antibiotic therapy is essential. Surgery is needed for perforation of the intestine or peritonitis. Dead bowel tissue is

(continued)

Table A.1 (continued)

Name	Description	Signs and symptoms	Treatment
	often seen in neonates who are ill or premature.		removed. The colostomy or ileostomy is reversed later.
Osmotic diarrhea	Results from too much water drawn into the bowel. Excessive intake of sugar, salt, or dietetic candy [due to sorbitol], or a wide variety of malabsorption disorders (e.g., see celiac disease, pancreatic diseases, lactose intolerance).	Excessive and frequent watery stools and bloating. Can include steatorrhea with fat digestion or malabsorption problems and sugar in the stool for carbohydrate digestion or malabsorption problems. Stool volume declines with fasting.	Avoid intake of offending dietary substance and/or treat the underlying digestive or malabsorption disease.
Pseudomembranous colitis	Inflammation of the colon associated with use of most antibiotics, except vancomycin, leading to overgrowth of *C. difficile* (see above).	Diarrhea can be watery and sometimes bloody accompanied by abdominal cramps and pain, fever, pus, or mucus in the stool, nausea, and dehydration. Shallow superficial ulcers can develop that are covered by neutrophils, fibrin, bacteria, or cellular debris.	Switching the antibiotic to vancomycin or others that are effective against *C. difficile*. Surgery for rupture of the intestinal wall or peritonitis. Fecal replacement therapy from a close relative or household member.
Secretory diarrhea	Results from increased active secretion of body water into the bowel or potentially an inhibition of water absorption. This can result from GI tract infections (e.g., *vibrio cholerae*, *E. coli*, *clostridium*), certain drugs, or other conditions (e.g., see VIPoma in Appendix Table B.1).	Excessive and frequent watery stools with a daily volume of more than one liter. The stool volume is unchanged with fasting unlike with osmotic diarrhea.	Treatment depends on the cause, age of the patient, extent of dehydration, and other factors. Many bacterial infections correct on their own while others, especially if serious, require antibiotics. Identification of the offending organism is essential.
Sodium–glucose linked transporter (SGLT1) deficiency	Lack of the transporter prevents absorption of dietary galactose and decreases absorption of dietary glucose though the latter can also be absorbed by the intestinal GLUT-5 transporter.	Osmotic diarrhea and an inability to properly process dietary lactose, the primary source of galactose.	Limiting lactose and specifically galactose in the diet.
Toxigenic diarrhea	Caused by the enterotoxins produced by enterotoxigenic bacteria such as *V. cholera* and the *E. coli* strains that are specifically enterotoxigenic.	Watery and voluminous diarrhea.	See specific bacterial infections above.
Traveler's diarrhea	GI disorder caused by consuming contaminated food or water when traveling to regions where climate, social	Loose stools, diarrhea, and abdominal cramps. Not a serious condition.	Antimotility agents, bismuth subsalicylate [Pepto-bismol] or antibiotics as appropriate.

(continued)

Table A.1 (continued)

Name	Description	Signs and symptoms	Treatment
	conditions, or sanitary standards differ from your normal. Most commonly caused by enterotoxigenic *E. coli* infection (see above).		
Trehalose intolerance	Inability to digest dietary trehalose because of deficiency of the brush border enzyme trehalase. Most common in Greenland and other Inuit populations.	Colonic bacteria process the trehalose producing gas accompanied by osmotic diarrhea (see above), bloating, and vomiting.	Avoid trehalose in the diet by eliminating the intake of edible mushrooms from the diet.
Tropical sprue (tropical diarrhea)	A malabsorption syndrome usually associated with gastroenteritis acquired in tropical or subtropical regions. Bacteria from those regions cause inflammation and damage to small intestine.	Diarrhea, which is worse on a high-fat diet, abdominal cramps, excessive gas, indigestion, muscle cramps, paleness, and weight loss are seen to varying degrees.	Treat dehydration or reduce potential for dehydration with fluids and electrolytes. Vitamin and mineral replacement specifically folate, iron, vitamin B_{12}, and fat soluble vitamins. For adults, tetracycline but not for children as it discolors teeth that are forming.
Ulcerative colitis	An inflammatory bowel disease that causes inflammation of the mucosa in the colon. The disease begins at the anal verge and extends proximally in a contiguous pattern unlike Crohn's disease that is associated with skip lesions. Extent of disease associated with cancer risk.	Features include bloody diarrhea, abdominal pain, weight loss, fever, loss of appetite, joint pain, nausea, and vomiting. In early stages massive hemorrhage, toxic megacolon, and perforation can occur. In later stages, strictures, colon cancer, and sclerosing cholangitis can occur.	Especially when confined to the anal verge or descending colon, topical agents (cortisone or mesalamine) via enema. A variety of oral agents can be used for more advanced disease. Surgery is reserved for severe complications or lack of response to medical therapy.
Whipple's disease	Infection by *Tropheryma whippeli* causing the lymphatic system associated with enterocytes to become blocked with fat due to reduced movement of chylomicrons to the thoracic duct. Blockage causes decreased fat absorption. Rare but most often seen in middle-aged white men.	Joint pain is commonly seen initially likely because of defective immune response that may make a patient susceptible to the initial infection. Additionally there is steatorrhea, diarrhea, weight loss, bloating, abdominal pain, fatigue, and anemia.	IV ceftriaxone followed by another antibiotic (e.g., trimethoprim-sulfamethoxazole) for up to 1 year.

Appendix B

Table B.1 Benign, premalignant, malignant growths and neoplasms affecting the GI tract and organs involved with digestion

Name	Description	Treatment
Oral cavity and salivary glands		
Acinic cell carcinoma	An uncommon salivary tumor, mostly (80 %) in the parotid but also the submandibular gland. It is sometimes bilateral and multicentric and asymptomatic in early stages. Symptoms can include enlarged salivary gland. More commonly found in women than men. The tumor can be solid, microcystic, trabecular, or follicular type.	Surgery often with postsurgery radiation; neutron beam radiation; conventional radiation; or chemotherapy.
Adenoid cystic carcinoma	Comprises 3–5 % of all and is the third most common malignant salivary gland tumor. Most occur in parotid but may also be in minor salivary glands. Generally a slow growing mass common in the fifth–seventh decades of life, often associated with pain and tenderness. The tumor exhibits cribiform, tubular, or solid patterns. Generally the solid patterns are a higher grade tumor. Perinuclear involvement also common.	Surgical removal with clean margins. Adjuvant or palliative radiotherapy usually follows surgery. Fast neutron therapy may be the most effective for inoperable or recurrent tumors. Chemotherapy used if tumor metastasizes.

(continued)

E. Trowers and M. Tischler, *Gastrointestinal Physiology*,
DOI 10.1007/978-3-319-07164-0, © Springer International Publishing Switzerland 2014

Table B.1 (continued)

Name	Description	Treatment
Erythroplakia	Oral lesions that appear as a flat red, velvety lesion (patch) often recur and are at high risk of carcinoma. Associated with tobacco use, persistent irritation, and human papilloma virus (HPV). Patients are usually 40–70 years of age.	Lesion is biopsied to determine extent of the dysplasia and may be completely excised depending on the finding.
Hairy leukoplakia	A benign growth associated with Epstein–Barr virus seen primarily in HIV-infected patients as well as immune-compromised patients. A low risk of carcinoma in this lesion. It appears as corrugated or hairy, white patches on the side of the tongue.	Treatment is not necessary. The condition may resolve with high doses of acyclovir.
Mucoepidermoid carcinoma	The most common malignant salivary gland tumors and the most common malignant salivary gland neoplasm in young (<20) patients. Mostly (60–70 %) in parotids. It presents as a painless enlargement of the parotid or submandibular gland for 1 year or less. Epithelial cells demonstrate mixture of squamous, intermediate, and mucus secreting cells; with a broad spectrum of differentiation. Low grade tumors tend to have predominantly mucus secreting cells forming glandular spaces, high grade tumors are largely squamous epithelial cells.	High grade tumors are treated aggressively using surgery. For low-grade tumors a partial or total laryngectomy may be recommended depending on the specific tumor location.
Squamous papilloma	Benign neoplasm of the oral epithelium; mostly on ventral tongue, palate, and mucosal surface of lips; associated with human papillomavirus (HPV). It is characterized by small finger-like projections causing a lesion with a rough or wart-like surface. It often has a white appearance.	Cured by excision; recurrence or appearance of new lesions suggests retransmission of the virus or possibly a carcinoma.

(continued)

Table B.1 (continued)

Name	Description	Treatment
Pleomorphic adenoma	The most common (50 %) tumor of major salivary glands and 60 % of all parotid tumors. It is a mixed tumor exhibiting both epithelial and mesenchymal differentiation. The tumor is encapsulated and lobulated. Microscopically epithelial cells appear as ducts or cords amid a matrix though there could also be little matrix.	Needle biopsy prior to surgery to confirm the diagnosis. Adjuvant radiotherapy may be used if the tumor is malignant.
Warthin tumor (papillary cystadenoma lymphomatosum)	A benign tumor primarily of the parotid salivary glands. The second most common salivary neoplasm especially in males 50–70 and smokers with an eightfold greater risk. Signs include swollen salivary gland; lump near back of lower jaw with pain; facial nerve paralysis, tinnitus. The tumor is well encapsulated; narrow cystic/clefts lined by two layers of epithelial cells.	Cured by excision
Esophagus		
Adenocarcinoma	More common in males than females (5:1) and in whites more so than blacks. Appears to arise from dysplasia of Barrett's esophagus (see Table A.1), invades adjacent structures, and metastases are via lymphatics. Overall prognosis is poor. Early lesions are composed of flat or raised patches of intact mucosa; nodular or mass lesions that may ulcerate and infiltrate are seen in advanced cancers. Symptoms include dysphagia, progressive weight loss, vomiting, and bleeding in advanced disease. Less than half the patients give a history of symptoms of reflux disease.	Treatment depends on the stage of the tumor. Chemoradiation followed by surgery is often used for stages I, II, or III.

(continued)

Table B.1 (continued)

Name	Description	Treatment
Squamous cell carcinoma	Invasive carcinoma linked to chronic inflammatory state due to dietary and/or environmental factors; most common in black males ($5\times$ in males; $4\times$ in blacks); onset above age 60. Symptoms include dysphagia and recent weight loss. The tumor is usually far advanced at diagnosis. Tracheal involvement associated with pneumonia or coughing due to mucus aspiration. Poor prognosis (5–10 % 5-year survival) with metastasis via lymphatics.	Surgery alone or chemotherapy and radiation combined with surgery.
Stomach		
Adenoma	Represent about 10 % of gastric tumors, vary in size and are usually found in the antrum. Risk of malignancy increases with polyp size. Microscopically composed of dysplastic epithelium similar to colon polyps. The neoplasm is circumscribed and composed of tubular and/or villous structures showing intraepithelial neoplasia.	Endoscopic mucosal resection— elevated lesion <2 cm; depressed lesion <1 cm. Endoscopic submucosal dissection used but a much more difficult procedure. Eradication of *H. pylori* in early neoplasms improves prognosis.
Adenocarcinoma	Variety of potential causal factors including *H. pylori* infection leading to chronic gastritis; comprises 95 % of gastric malignancies. Asymptomatic in early stages and later symptoms include weight loss, abdominal pain, anorexia, chronic blood loss. Invades stomach wall and is a flat or excavated lesion often in cardia, body, and fundus of stomach. Prognosis is less than 15 % for a 5-year survival.	Surgical procedure depends on size and location; often includes lymphadenectomy due to metastasis via lymphatics to lymph nodes, liver, and other distant sites.

(continued)

Table B.1 (continued)

Name	Description	Treatment
Carcinoid tumors	These malignant gastric tumors are rare (3 % of total gastric malignancies). They arise from epithelial neuroendocrine cells. They exist as multiple small lesions. Symptoms generally do not appear unless the tumor metastasizes to the liver and then symptoms are more likely with intestinal carcinoids. The tumor produces hormone-like substances. Prognosis is only 20 % 5-year survival when it metastasizes. (see also Zollinger–Ellison syndrome.)	Proton pump inhibitor (omeprazole) may be used as a short-term treatment at a low dosage. Standard treatments include surgery, radiotherapy, interferons, and somatostatin analogues.
Leiomyomas; leiomyoblastomas	A rare, benign mesenchymal gastric tumor most commonly found in males 50–70. Usually located in the corpus of the stomach but also the antrum and may protrude into the mucosa. Patients remain asymptomatic for long periods of time. Eventually symptoms might include bleeding or ulceration.	Treatment is surgical resection.
Lipoma	A benign tumor usually in the antrum of the stomach. Usually in the submucosa and occur singly. The most common presentation is bleeding due to ulceration.	Treatment is surgical resection.
Lymphoma	Patients with *H. pylori* gastritis have an increased risk of a gastric lymphoma. Most are non-Hodgkin type and are of the mucosa-associated lymphoid tissue. In early stages, patients are asymptomatic. Common later symptoms are nonspecific.	Treatments shifted from surgery to chemotherapy and *H. pylori* antibiotic eradication. Radiotherapy may be used if antibiotic therapy fails to yield improvement.
Pancreas		
Congenital cysts	Most cysts are multiple, and associated with underlying congenital diseases that primarily affect other organ systems. Solitary congenital cysts are rare. Result from anomalous development of the pancreatic ducts. They are unilocular, thin walled, and up to 5 cm in diameter. Cysts are lined by	Generally these cysts are locally excised.

(continued)

Table B.1 (continued)

Name	Description	Treatment
	uniform cuboidal epithelium and are enclosed by a thin fibrous capsule filled with clear serous fluid. They appear sporadically.	
Ductal carcinoma	Most common (85 %) type of cancer of the pancreas and the fourth leading cause of cancer deaths in men and women in the USA. Risk factors include smoking, diets high in fats and red meat, and chronic pancreatitis (see table on GI diseases). Early disease usually does not exhibit symptoms and when they do appear is generally nonspecific and varied. The mortality rate is high with <5 % 5-year survival with many dying within 6 months after diagnosis.	The tumor in fewer than half of patients is contained entirely within the pancreas at diagnosis. In these patients, surgical excision is recommended providing the best option for long-term survival.
Intraductal papillary mucinous neoplasm	A mucin-producing intraductal neoplasm generally found in the head of the pancreas occurring more often in men and 10–20 % is multifocal. They often involve a larger pancreatic duct.	Treatment is surgical resection with evaluation for invasive malignancy.
Pseudocyst	Localized collections of necrotic–hemorrhagic material rich in pancreatic enzymes. They lack an epithelial lining ("pseudo") and are large; up to 30 cm in diameter. They are common (~75 % of pancreatic cysts) and linked to alcohol abuse and trauma. They are typically solitary and may be within the pancreatic parenchyma. Expansion can result in abdominal pain, duodenal or biliary obstruction, vascular occlusion, or fistula formation into adjacent viscera, the pleural space or pericardium. They may cause spontaneous infection, pancreatic ascites, or pleural effusion.	A variety of treatments are available for pseudocysts. The treatment is complex and a multidisciplinary team of experienced pancreatic surgeon, gastroenterologist, and radiologist working together.

(continued)

Table B.1 (continued)

Name	Description	Treatment
Serous cystadenoma	Benign cystic neoplasm accounting for 25 % of such neoplasms in the pancreas. Occurs twice as often in women in the seventh decade of life, usually presenting due to abdominal pain or mass. The neoplasm consists of glycogen-rich cuboidal cells lining small (1–3 mm) cysts containing clear fluid.	Surgical resection is curative.
Verner–Morrison syndrome (VIPoma)	An endocrine tumor, originating from non-beta islet cells, that produces vasoactive intestinal peptide (VIP) and may be associated with multiple endocrine neoplasia type 1. The massive amount of VIP causes chronic watery diarrhea leading to dehydration, hypokalemia, achlorhydria, acidosis, vasodilation (flushing and hypotension), hypercalcemia, and hyperglycemia.	Dehydration corrected with IV fluids to replace those lost in diarrhea. Drugs slow the diarrhea (e.g., octreotide blocks VIP action). The best chance of a cure is surgical excision of the tumor prior to metastasis.
Zollinger–Ellison syndrome	An endocrine tumor of non-beta islet cells that secretes gastrin, which stimulates acid secreting cells of the stomach. Excessive acid production leads to ulceration. It may be associated with multiple endocrine neoplasia type 1. Symptoms can include chronic diarrhea, steatorrhea, esophageal pain, vomiting digested blood, and weight loss due to decreased appetite.	Can be surgically excised or treated with chemotherapy. Symptoms treated with both proton pump inhibitors (e.g., omeprazole) and antagonists of histamine-2 receptors (e.g., famotidine) to slow acid secretion. Octreotide seems the best drug for overall medical treatment.
Liver and hepatic bile ducts		
Adenoma	A benign tumor. Bile duct adenomas are rarely over 1 cm and usually incidental. Liver cell adenomas typically occur in young women with oral contraceptive use. They are 1–2 cm up to 30 cm, yellow-tan, frequently bile stained, nodular, and soft with prominent vascularity and	The adenoma should be resected as long as it is surgically accessible. Patients should avoid oral contraceptives and hormone replacement therapy.

(continued)

Table B.1 (continued)

Name	Description	Treatment
	no bile duct structure. About 25–50 % cause pain in the right upper quadrant or epigastric region of the abdomen. Since they can be large, patients may notice a palpable mass. Usually they are asymptomatic, and may be discovered incidentally on imaging ordered for some unrelated reason. If not treated, there is a risk of bleeding that can lead to hypotension, tachycardia, and sweating (diaphoresis).	
Cholangiocarcinoma	Composed of mutated epithelial cells (or cells showing characteristics of epithelial differentiation) that originate in the bile ducts that drain bile from the liver. A relatively rare neoplasm. Signs and symptoms include abnormal liver function tests, abdominal pain, jaundice, and weight loss; changes in color of stool or urine may also occur. Known risk factors include primary sclerosing cholangitis (see table on GI diseases), congenital liver malformations, infection with parasitic liver flukes, or exposure to Thorotrast. Most patients have no identifiable specific risk factors.	Treatment depends on the size and location of the tumor, whether it has spread, and the patient's overall health. The only effective treatments are surgical resection or liver transplant because the tumor is aggressive. There is no effective medical treatment.
Metastatic tumor	They are produced by metastasis of cancer from other tissues. The liver is a common site for their appearance because of its rich blood supply from the hepatic artery and portal vein. Half of all cases metastasize from the GI tract but also from breast, ovaries, lung, and kidney. Imaging appearances of liver metastases are nonspecific. Biopsy specimens are used for histologic diagnosis. Symptoms may be lacking but can include pain in the upper right quadrant, jaundice, or nausea.	Metastatic nature of the disease often requires whole body chemotherapy. Surgical resection of the tumor depends on size and location. Radiotherapy may also be used.

(continued)

Table B.1 (continued)

Name	Description	Treatment
Gallbladder		
Adenoma	Most common benign epithelial tumor of gallbladder similar to those elsewhere in the GI tract; found in <1 % of cholecystectomy specimens. Not a premalignant lesion since molecular abnormalities differ from carcinoma. A 3–25 mm polypoid structure projecting into the gallbladder lumen may be sessile and the vast majority (90 %) are single. Familial adenomatous polyposis and Peutz–Jeghers syndrome (see below) are associated with an increased prevalence of adenomas of the gallbladder and biliary tract. Adenomas are usually asymptomatic and discovered incidentally during radiologic evaluation for abdominal pain. There may be chronic or intermittent right upper quadrant pain.	Treatment is total surgical excision.
Carcinoma: extrahepatic bile ducts	Typically found in elderly patients presenting with painless jaundice with a slight male predominance. Risk factors include biliary tree fluke infections, primary sclerosing cholangitis, IBD, and choledochal cysts. Symptoms include painless jaundice, nausea, vomiting, weight loss; hepatomegaly in about 50 % of patients and less frequently with a palpable gallbladder. The prognosis is poor; mean survival 6–18 months. The tumor appears as firm gray nodules within the bile duct wall. The infiltration type may cause diffuse thickening of the gallbladder wall and present with extensive fibrosis accompanying epithelial proliferation.	Surgery of the bile duct with partial hepatectomy as needed, and/or the Whipple procedure. If tumor cannot be removed but blocks the small intestine causing bile to build up in the gallbladder, biliary bypass may be done. Radiation therapy and/or chemotherapy may also be used depending on the situation.

(continued)

Table B.1 (continued)

Name	Description	Treatment
Carcinoma: gallbladder	A slight female predominance of this tumor most commonly appearing in the seventh decade. Gallstones and/or infection may be risk factors. Symptoms are similar to cholelithiasis including right upper quadrant pain and jaundice. Usually the tumor is an incidental finding at surgery; most invade the liver. The tumor can show two patterns of growth; infiltrating with irregular, diffuse thickening of the gallbladder wall that grossly feels firm or exophytic with an irregular, cauliflower-like mass growing into the gallbladder lumen and invading the underlying wall. These are usually adenocarcinoma and rarely squamous or carcinoid. Prognosis is very poor with just 1 % 5-year survival.	Three types of treatment: surgery, chemotherapy, and radiation therapy. Surgery involves cholecystectomy with removal of nearby lymph nodes and sometimes part of the liver. If the tumor cannot be removed, palliative surgery may relieve symptoms.
Choledochal cysts	Congenital dilatations of the common bile duct. Cysts are at risk for developing into bile duct carcinoma. Uncommon in Western countries and most present in the first year of life. Adult presentation is rare but at that stage is associated with complication. The classic triad of symptoms found in a minority of patients includes intermittent abdominal pain, jaundice, and a right upper quadrant abdominal mass.	Surgical excision of the cyst.
Inflammatory polyps	Benign mucosal projections lined by columnar epithelium, with a central stromal core infiltrated by chronic inflammatory cells and lipid-laden macrophages. They appear as either sessile or pedunculated, and are composed of fibrous and granulation tissue. Polyps usually 5–10 mm in size but can exceed 1 cm. Larger polyps can be confused with a carcinoma. Most are nonneoplastic and rarely cause symptoms.	Cholecystectomy suggested for larger polyps due to increased risk of adenoma or carcinoma. Smaller polyps are monitored for future growth to a large polyp.

(continued)

Table B.1 (continued)

Name	Description	Treatment
Intestine (small and large)		
Adenoma	Benign tumors that may have a stalk or be broad based (sessile); three types are tubular (75 %), tubulovillous, and villous. Tubular arise in the rectosigmoid region generally in older males (average 60) and often pedunculated. Appear as closely spaced glands with crowded cells, decreased mucin production, and "migration" of nuclei from basal position in gland. Adenomas have a very low risk of carcinoma. Tubulovillous have hybrid features of tubular and villous adenomas; risk of carcinoma increases with more villus features. Villus adenomas have greater than 50 % villus features. Patient age usually 60–65 with the site most often being rectosigmoid. Tumors are usually sessile and frond-like; fronds are composed of connective tissue core covered by colonic epithelium.	Treatment is endoscopic/surgical excision.
Adenocarcinoma	Though uncommon in the small intestine, when present the duodenum is most commonly involved. Increased risk in patients with celiac disease, Crohn's (see Table A.1), Peutz–Jeghers syndrome (see below), or familial adenomatous polyposis (see below). Tumors may appear annular or as a polypoid mass. Symptoms include nausea, bloating, weight loss, obstruction, jaundice, iron deficiency anemia, and fatigue. Prognosis is poor with a 5-year survival of <35 %.	Treatment consists of surgical resection and or chemoradiation therapy.
Carcinoid syndrome	See carcinoid tumor	

(continued)

Table B.1 (continued)

Name	Description	Treatment
Carcinoid tumor	The majority (~40 %) occur in the small intestine arising from neuroendocrine cells and usually in older patients (>50 years). Symptoms reflect the hormones produced by the tumor. Intestinal carcinoid syndrome is associated with serotonin secretion as well as histamine and bradykinin. Carcinoid syndrome is characterized by diarrhea, cutaneous flushing, sweating, bronchospasm, colicky abdominal pain, and right-sided cardiac valvular fibrosis. When confined to the intestine, the serotonin released into the blood is metabolized by the liver and hence is usually associated with tumor metastasis to the liver. The tumors appear as mucosal or submucosal nodules with yellow coloration. The tumor cells are small and uniform with "salt and pepper" chromatin and may be arranged in nests or cords.	Standard treatment can include surgery, chemotherapy, radiation therapy, or hormone therapy. Hormone therapy with a somatostatin analogue stops extra hormones from being made by the tumor.
Familial adenomatous polyposis (FAP)	Mutation occurs in the adenomatous polyposis coli gene. Diagnosis requires at least 100 polyps (classic) to be present. Single polyps have similar features as sporadic adenoma. Associated with extraintestinal manifestations. Colorectal adenocarcinoma develops in all patients if left untreated. Symptoms may include bleeding from the rectum, change in bowel habits, abdominal pain, low blood counts, or unexplained weight loss.	Colectomy is the treatment of choice.
Gardner's syndrome (familial colorectal polyposis; FCP)	An autosomal dominant form of polyposis characterized by the presence of multiple polyps in the colon together with tumors outside the colon.	Sulindac, an indomethacin derivative produces regression of polyps in 80 % of cases of familial adenomatous polyposis, after total colectomy.

(continued)

Table B.1 (continued)

Name	Description	Treatment
Hamartomatous polyps	Nonneoplastic tumor-like growth of mature tissues normally present at the site in which they occur, usually as a genetically determined polyposis syndrome due to faulty development. Grow at the normal rate of the host tissue rarely causing problems. A common example is a strawberry naevus. Often found by chance as usually are asymptomatic, though rectal bleeding and bloody stools can occur.	Polyps can be removed during a colonoscopy or sigmoidoscopy.
Hereditary nonpolyposis colorectal cancer (Lynch syndrome; HNCC)	A mutation of the DNA mismatch repair gene. Lesions are sessile with serrated and mucinous features. Colon cancers tend to occur on the right side in younger patients. Colorectal adenocarcinoma develops in the majority of patients and associated with other malignancies including in the stomach and small intestine. Individuals have ~80 % lifetime risk for colon cancer. Early states are usually asymptomatic. In later stages symptoms include rectal bleeding, change in bowel habits, change in stool size (possibly due to obstruction), and significant weight loss.	Chemotherapy with segmental tumor resection is the treatment of choice.
Hyperplastic polyps	Common polyps often routinely found during a colonoscopy. They are benign and share similar features to a sessile serrated adenoma but unlike adenomas do not exhibit dysplasia making progress to colorectal cancer less likely.	The usual treatment is removal by polypectomy, laparotomy, or complete resection.
Juvenile polyposis syndrome (JPS)	Results from a mutation in either of two genes and appears in children younger than 5. Malformations of mucosal epithelium and lamina propria occur with most located in the rectum leading to rectal bleeding. Also associated with increased risk of other GI	Yearly upper and lower endoscopies with polyp excision and cytology may be necessary. Malignant transformation of polyps requires surgical colectomy.

(continued)

Table B.1 (continued)

Name	Description	Treatment
	malignancies in stomach, small intestine, colon, and pancreas. Occurrence in infancy is the most severe form of the disorder with the poorest outcome. This condition results in severe diarrhea, failure to thrive, and cachexia.	
Lymphomatous polyps	A rare GI non-Hodgkin lymphoma forming numerous polyps. Patients predominantly male, 40–80. Generally polyps occur at multiple sites from esophagus to rectum with multiple polyps that may aggregate. Most cases are due to mantle cell lymphoma. The lymphomatous infiltrate predominantly involves the submucosa and lamina propria.	Treatment involves surgical removal.
Lynch syndrome	See hereditary nonpolyposis colorectal cancer.	
Peutz–Jeghers syndrome	Inherited (autosomal dominant) disorder associated with development of intestinal polyps creating a high risk for cancer (cumulative risk 39 % colon; 13 % small intestine). Melanin pigmentation appears on lips, gums, inner lining of mouth, skin. The patient may have clubbed fingers or toes, abdominal cramping pain, bloody stool, or vomiting.	Numerous surgeries to remove polyps causing long-term problems; iron supplements due to blood loss; frequent monitoring for cancerous polyp changes.

Appendix C

Table C.1 Clinical laboratory tests

Test	Description	Normal range of values[a]
Complete blood count (CBC)		
Hemoglobin (Hb or Hgb)	Hb contained in red blood cells (RBC) carries O_2 to body tissues and aids in returning CO_2 to lungs. Hb is measured by an automated analyzer after changing to cyanomethemoglobin whose color can be quantitated. EDTA (calcium chelator) containing tubes prevent coagulation. High levels of lipids, serum protein, immunoglobulins, fibrinogen, bilirubin, or white blood cells (WBC) can cause erroneous elevations.	Male: 13.8–17.2 g/dL Female: 12.0–15.6 g/dL
Hematocrit (Hct)	The proportion of blood volume taken up by RBCs. A blood sample in a capillary tube is centrifuged. The height of the packed RBCs and of the column of blood is measured. Hct is calculated as the packed RBC height × 100 divided by the column of blood height.	Male: 41–52 % Female: 35–47 % Result is usually about three times the Hb value
Red blood cells (RBC)	RBCs are the most common blood cell. The test indicates the number per volume. When abnormal RBCs are present, microscopic examination is required to evaluate and describe their numbers and morphology.	Male: 4.4–$5.8 \times 10^6/\mu L$ Female: 3.9–$5.2 \times 10^6/\mu L$

(continued)

E. Trowers and M. Tischler, *Gastrointestinal Physiology*,
DOI 10.1007/978-3-319-07164-0, © Springer International Publishing Switzerland 2014

Table C.1 (continued)

Test	Description	Normal range of values[a]
Erythrocyte sedimentation rate (ESR)	The rate at which RBCs sediment in 1 h. The ESR indirectly measures inflammation reflecting the balance between factors promoting the sedimentation of RBCs and those opposing. ESR can be altered in some disorders but can also be heightened in situations such as pregnancy.	Male: $\leq$20 mm/h
	Correction for age may be used: $\leq$[Age (years) + 10 (female)] $\times$ 0.5.	Female: $\leq$30 mm/h
Mean corpuscular volume (MCV)	Measure of the average RBC size. MCV is calculated as the Hct (%) $\times$ 10 divided by total number of RBCs.	80–100 fL
Mean corpuscular hemoglobin (MCH)	Measure of the average mass of Hb per RBC in a sample of blood. MCH is calculated as : total mass of Hb $\times$ 10 divided by number of RBCs.	26–34 pg/cell
Mean corpuscular hemoglobin concentration (MCHC)	The concentration of Hb within a certain volume of red blood cells. MCHC is calculated as the amount of Hb divided by Hct.	32–36 g/dL
Red blood cell distribution width (RDW)	A measure of the variance of the width of RBC. Width is directly related to the volume. Higher values indicate greater size variation. RDW is calculated as the MCV standard deviation per mL blood divided by the average MCV.	6–8 μm
Reticulocytes	Count of immature RBCs. They develop and mature in bone marrow but circulate about 1 day before maturing.	0.5–2.3 % of total RBCs
White blood cells (leukocytes; WBC)	Cells of the immune system that fight infectious disease and foreign substances. There are 5 types [described below] that include neutrophils, lymphocytes, monocytes eosinophils, and basophils.	$3.8–10.8 \times 10^3$/μL Differential: Neutrophil: 1,500–7,800/μL Lymphocyte: 850–4,100/μL Monocyte: 200–1,100/μL Eosinophil: 50–1,500/μL Basophil: 0–200/μL

(continued)

Table C.1 (continued)

Test	Description	Normal range of values[a]
Neutrophil granuloctyes	Most abundant white blood cell in mammals. Referred to as neutrophils or polymorphonuclear neutrophils (PMNs).	See differential under WBC
Lymphocytes	WBC in the immune system. Large lymphocytes include natural killer (NK) cells. Small lymphocytes include T cells and B cells.	See differential under WBC
Monocytes	WBC in the innate immune system of vertebrates that play multiple functions including replenishing macrophages; in response to inflammation move to site of infection. Half are stored in the spleen.	See differential under WBC
Eosinophilic granulocytes	Usually called eosinophils and less often acidophils. They combat multicellular parasites and certain infections and also control mechanisms associated with asthma and allergic reactions.	See differential under WBC
Basophilic granulocytes	Usually called basophils. These are the least common of the WBC.	See differential under WBC
Platelets	Aid in the formation of blood clots. Automatically determined with particle counting techniques based on proprietary electrical impedance or optical methods.	150–$450 \times 10^3/\mu L$
Comprehensive metabolic panel (CMP)		
Albumin	The most plentiful protein in the serum and secreted by the liver. Chronic liver disease lowers its blood amount. Measured colorimetrically by binding to bromocresol green dye. Comparison to standards allows determination of albumin concentration.	3.5–5.0 g/dL
Alkaline phosphatase (ALP)	Elevated as a result of damage to bile ducts (e.g., obstruction due to gallstones). Normally measured by production of yellow-colored 4-nitrophenoxide from colorless 4-nitrophenol phosphate substrate in the presence of ALP.	40–120 U/L Bone isozyme: 0–55 U/L Liver isozyme: 0–94 U/L
Alanine aminotransferase (ALT; also SGPT)	Elevation in the serum (along with AST, below) is used to assess liver damage though ALT is also found in smaller amounts in other tissues (e.g., kidney, muscle). ALT catalyzes the reaction: alanine	Male: 0–35 U/L Female: 0–20 U/L AST/ALT > 2 generally reflects severe liver damage due to chronic alcoholism or other major chronic liver disease.

(continued)

Table C.1 (continued)

Test	Description	Normal range of values[a]
	$+ \alpha$-ketoglutarate $\rightleftharpoons$ pyruvate $+$ glutamate and is monitored indirectly by production of pyruvate or glutamate products via a coupled, enzyme reaction that results in a colored or other measurable product.	
Aspartate aminotransferase (AST; also sGOT)	Its elevation in the serum (along with ALT, above) is used to assess liver damage though AST is also reasonably abundant in other tissues (e.g., kidney, muscle, heart, pancreas). AST catalyzes the reaction aspartate $+$ α-ketoglutarate $\rightleftharpoons$ oxaloacetate $+$ glutamate and is monitored indirectly by the production of either oxaloacetate or glutamate products via a coupled, enzyme reaction that results in a colored or other measurable product.	Male: 0–37 U/L Female: 0–31 U/L AST/ALT > 2 generally reflects severe liver damage due to chronic alcoholism or other major chronic liver disease.
Bicarbonate/carbon dioxide (CO_2)	Bicarbonate is an important biological blood buffer. In response to metabolic acidosis, the concentration decreases due to rapid respiration to expire CO_2 that reduces the acid load $[H^+ + HCO_3^- \rightarrow CO_2 + H_2O]$. Normally measured as total CO_2 [~95 % bicarbonate plus ~5 % dissolved CO_2 plus carbonic acid]. Measured by acid liberation of CO_2 that reacts with a bicarbonate–carbonate buffer with an indicator dye and calibrated with a known standard.	22–29 mEq/L
Bilirubin	Derived from breakdown of heme in Hb when RBCs turnover. Total bilirubin includes an insoluble form (nonconjugated) derived directly from heme and a soluble form that is conjugated with glucuronic acid in the liver. Determined by an azo dye producing a red-violet azobilirubin. Ethanol is added to the test sample prior to the dye so that both conjugated (direct) and unconjugated (indirect) bilirubin react to provide the total bilirubin value.	Total: <0.1–1.3 mg/dL Conjugated: <0.4 mg/dL

(continued)

Table C.1 (continued)

Test	Description	Normal range of values[a]
Blood urea nitrogen (BUN)	Reflects the amount of nitrogen in the blood in the form of urea, which is excreted by kidneys. Along with creatinine (see below) when elevated is indicative of diminished kidney function. Normally measured by production of a yellow product. For more specific measurement the production of ammonia and carbonic acid from urea by the enzyme urease is determined spectrophotometrically by reaction of NH_3 with α-ketoglutaric acid.	7–30 mg/dL
Calcium (Ca^{2+})	Calcium plays an important role as a signal for cellular events by moving into and out of cells, as well as intracellular organelles. Normally measured utilizing colorimetric methods. Difficult to measure accurately due to false elevation in certain patients and under certain conditions (e.g., samples with hemolysis, high lipids, or abnormal albumin concentration), changes in plasma protein due to disease, exercise, sample acquisition, and dietary intake of calcium.	Serum: 8.5–10.3 mg/dL Ionized (serum): 4.5–5.6 mg/dL Urine: <300 mg/day
Chloride (Cl^-)	Important in cell metabolism and acid–base balance. Normally measured by reaction with mercuric thiocyanate. Thiocyanate reacts with ferric ions (Fe^{3+}) to form a compound whose concentration can be measured spectrophotometrically, allowing quantitative determination.	95–108 mEq/L
Creatinine	The breakdown product of creatine primarily found in skeletal muscle provides a measure of decreased kidney function. Usually measured by formation of a red-colored complex between creatine and alkaline picrate.	0.7–1.4 mg/dL

(continued)

Table C.1 (continued)

Test	Description	Normal range of values[a]
Glucose	The conversion of glucose, water, and oxygen to gluconic acid and hydrogen peroxide via glucose oxidase forms the basis for most clinical laboratory and home-based determinations of glucose. Further oxidation and color change of a reporter molecule by the hydrogen peroxide or measurement of oxygen consumption allows quantitation of glucose concentration. Whole blood values are lower than serum or plasma.	Fasting: 80–120 mg/dL
Potassium (K^+)	Important in brain and nerve function as well as maintaining osmotic balance. Most is intracellular and is maintained by the exchange of blood potassium for cell sodium via the Na^+/K^+-ATPase pump. Measured using an ion-specific electrode that is permeable to potassium.	3.5–5.0 mEq/L
Sodium (Na^+)	Sodium is essential for regulating blood volume, blood pressure, osmotic balance, and pH. Primarily found in the blood and is secreted from cells via the Na^+/K^+-ATPase pump. Measured using an ion-specific electrode that is permeable to sodium.	135–145 mEq/L
Total protein	The two major serum proteins are albumin (secreted by liver) and globulins (made by liver or immune system). Measured colorimetrically including the predominant protein albumin. A subset is determination of total globulin that is calculated by subtracting albumin from total protein.	Serum: 6.0–8.5 g/dL Urine: <150 mg/day
Other tests		
Thyroid hormones	Thyroxine (T4) and triiodothyronine (T3) are tyrosine-derived hormones. T4 is made in the thyroid follicular cell whereas most T3 is produced from T4 in peripheral cells. Though T4 is most abundant, T3 is much more potent and hence the primary thyroid hormone of biological action. The vast majority of circulating	T4 (total): 60–160 nmol/L T4 (free): 10–23 pmol/L T3 (total): 0.9–1.3 nmol/L T3 (free): 3.5–6.5 pmol/L

(continued)

Table C.1 (continued)

Test	Description	Normal range of values[a]
	thyroid hormone is protein bound. Only the free form is physiologically important. Thyroid hormones increase body energy consumption by elevating the activity of a variety of hormones that use energy such as the Na^+/K^+-ATPase pump.	
Thyroid stimulating hormone (TSH)	Secreted by the thyrotrophs of the anterior pituitary gland in response to a hypothalamic signal (thyrotropin-releasing hormone; TRH). TSH stimulates the thyroid follicular cell to synthesize and secrete thyroid hormone; mostly T4. TSH is the most sensitive indicator of thyroid function.	0.5–4.70 mIU/L

[a]Normal values: GlobalRPh. The clinician's ultimate reference. http://www.globalrph.com/labs_home.htm

g/dL = grams per 100 mL

mg/dL = 10^{-3} grams (milligrams) per 100 mL

pg = 10^{-12} grams; picogram

fL = 10^{-15} L

µL = 10^{-6} L; microliter = mm^3

Index